Seventh Edition

DIMENSIONS OF FOOD

Vickie A. Vaclavik, Ph.D., R.D.
University of Texas
Southwestern Medical Center
Dallas

Marcia H. Pimentel, M.S.
Senior Lecturer, Retired
Cornell University
Ithaca, New York

Marjorie M. Devine, Ph.D.
Professor Emeritus
Cornell University
Ithaca, New York

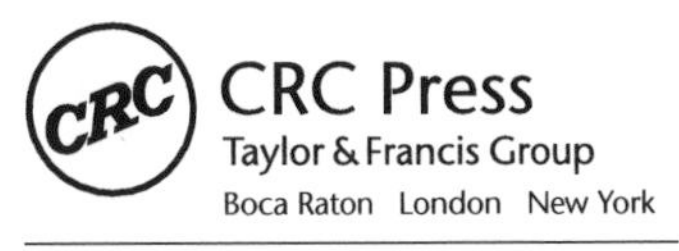

CRC Press
Taylor & Francis Group
Boca Raton London New York

CRC Press is an imprint of the
Taylor & Francis Group, an **informa** business

CRC Press
Taylor & Francis Group
6000 Broken Sound Parkway NW, Suite 300
Boca Raton, FL 33487-2742

Printed in the United States of America on acid-free paper
10 9 8 7 6 5 4 3 2 1

International Standard Book Number: 978-1-4398-2167-1 (Paperback)

Library of Congress Cataloging-in-Publication Data

Vaclavik, Vickie.
Dimensions of food / Vickie A. Vaclavik, Marcia H. Pimentel, Marjorie M. Devine. -- 7th ed.
p. cm.
Includes bibliographical references.
ISBN 978-1-4398-2167-1 (alk. paper)
1. Food--Laboratory manuals. 2. Nutrition--Laboratory manuals. 3. Cookery--Laboratory manuals. I. Pimentel, Marcia. H. II. Devine, Marjorie M. III. Title.

TX354.V33 2010
641.5--dc22 2009032043

Visit the Taylor & Francis Web site at
http://www.taylorandfrancis.com

and the CRC Press Web site at
http://www.crcpress.com

CONTENTS

PART III. HEATING FOODS BY MICROWAVE

PART IV. MEAL MANAGEMENT

Appendices

Preface

The whole world is in the food business—
at least in the consuming end.

— Irma Rombauer

Here is ***Dimensions of Food***, Seventh Edition—my, how time flies! This laboratory manual began as pages of student handouts printed in the purple ink of a well-used mimeograph machine at Cornell University. Today, this manual continues its original purpose of allowing students to explore the various dimensions of food—viewing economic, nutritional, palatability, chemical, sanitary, and food processing aspects of food.

Then, following the important chapters on the various dimensions of food, food principles are subsequently addressed by food item category, including:

- cereal and starch
- fruits and vegetables
- meat, poultry, and fish
- plant proteins
- eggs
- milk
- fats and oils
- sugars and sweeteners
- batters and dough

Each chapter contains ***Objectives, References, Assigned Readings, Terms, Exercises, and Recipes. Palatability Terms*** to use in reporting data are also included. Learning experiences move from basic demonstration to application. Throughout this manual, physical and chemical, functional and structural properties of food components are discussed in the chapter exercises. Study questions and problems are designed to assist students in clarifying and organizing facts into working principles. The questions cover the many dimensions of food—economic, nutritional, including food allergies, and so forth.

A section on microwave cooking and another on meal planning and preparation are included. Unique to this lab manual are extensive appendices. For example, in this seventh edition there is a new appendix dedicated to food allergies.

More than ever, students desire to be knowledgeable regarding what is ***in*** their food, how to make nutritious, safe food more convenient to prepare, and how to eat well on a budget! Therefore, the intent of this introductory foods manual is to involve students in a semester-long experience that provides them with a better understanding of food. Each food chapter closes with a ***Dietitian's Note***.

Our desire is to provide a variety of experiences from which instructors may choose those most helpful to their students. Space has been allocated for insertion of additional, teacher-provided material. As in the past, this manual is adaptable to two one-and-a-half-hour labs, or one three-hour lab; parts may be completed as independent study projects, with activities carried out in the lab or outside the classroom.

In keeping with the intent to better understand foods, once the exercises in this book have been completed, the student will have a personal and professional reference. Once again, as in earlier editions, we say "Thank you" to our students, whose curiosity and penetrating questions ***continue*** to make teaching the dimensions of food a joyful challenge!

V.A. Vaclavik
M.H. Pimentel
M.M. Devine

PART I

Dimensions of Food

Ah! Good eating is our goal, both personally and professionally. We desire that foods maximize our health and pleasure, and that food is nutritious, safe to eat, personally satisfying, and obtainable within the resources that each of us chooses to expend. Yet, realizing these goals in the marketplace is a challenge, a challenge of values, resources, choices, and conflicting information.

Today we have numerous suppliers from whom we can purchase various foods. However, we may hear or read conflicting nutrition-related news reports—even in the same day, causing us to become uncertain in our decisions about food. In the end, perhaps we are limited in our knowledge of exactly WHAT to purchase or exactly WHAT to think about good eating!

Part I of this manual helps clarify and examine in some depth the multidimensional nature of food decisions. Exercises, charts, and questions help investigate the economic, nutritional, palatability, sanitary, chemical, and processing dimensions of our food supply. Key principles are organized. Thus the relative values of food can be appraised and food choices tailored to the student's personal resources, needs, and beliefs.

Let's get started!

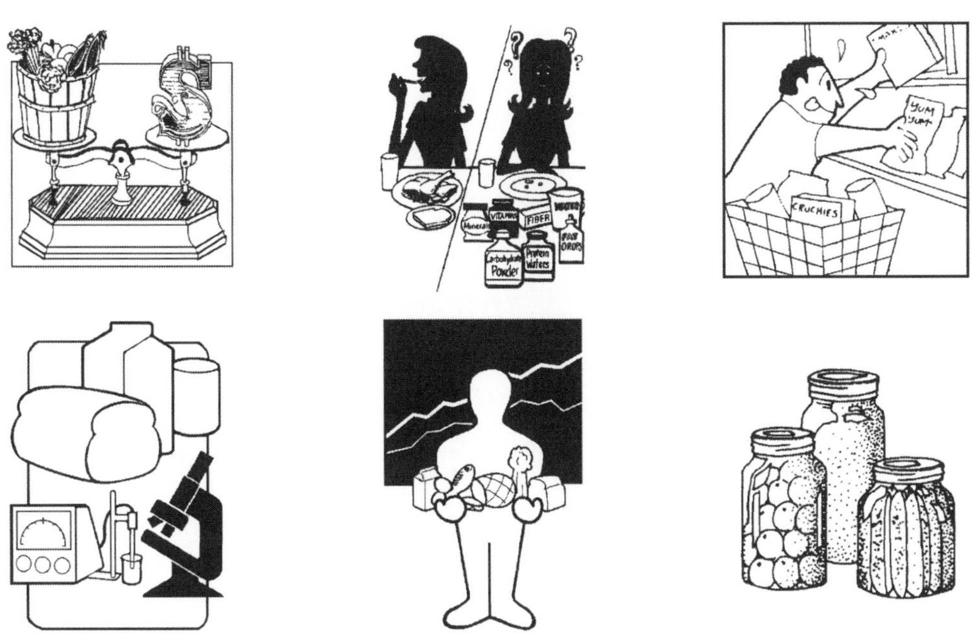

A. Economic Dimensions

He who steals my money gets trash;
he who steals my food gets a good meal!

— **Anonymous**

Objectives

To recognize factors that influence cost of food items
To calculate and compare cost per unit of various food items
To identify types of information available to the consumer in the marketplace
To delineate uses of different food qualities for specific purposes
To interpret, evaluate, and use food label information as a buying guide
To distinguish and enumerate the many considerations involved in choosing a "best food buy" for an individual or family

References[1]

Appendix A: Legislation Governing the Food Supply
Label Information to download: http://www.cfsan.fda.gov/~dms/foodlab.html#see1

Terms

Food, Drug and Cosmetic Act	Generic brand	A.P./E.P.
Food Additive Amendment	House brand	Unit pricing
Delaney Clause	NAS/NRC	Gross weight
Fair Packaging Act	RDA	Net weight
Labeling regulation	Daily value	Nutrition facts
Standards of identity	Dietary guidelines	"Planned-overs"

[1] Websites current at time of printing.

In the following sections, exercises are presented to illustrate some factors that affect the economy of food and food decisions. The exercises may be completed in the laboratory, as a class at a grocery store, or independently.

EXERCISE 1: FACTORS INFLUENCING THE COST OF FOOD

PROCEDURE

1. Complete the tables by matching the samples of products displayed with the price/item *or* independently, by visiting a grocery market.
2. Compare information and explanations with your classmates.

A. QUALITY OF PRODUCT—COMPARING STORE AND NATIONAL BRANDS

Brand	Price/Product	Price/Serving	Description	Uses of Product
National brand #1				
National brand #2				
Store brand				

1. Why is there a difference in *price per can* of the same product?

2. What is the difference between a store brand and a national brand?

3. What do the different labels state concerning the type of pack and net contents?

4. Which do you consider the "best buy"? What criteria are used by consumers in selecting canned products?

B. Caloric and Price Differences of Various Product Formulations

Evaluate the relative caloric and price differences among the regular and diet products, for example, canned fruit, salad dressings, soft drinks, etc.

Brand and Product	Calories/Serving	Cost/Serving
1 a. (reg.)		
b. (diet)		
2 a.		
b.		
3 a.		
b.		

1. Does the caloric value justify the price of any of these products? Explain.

2. How do caloric information and unit pricing assist in the consumer's food purchasing selection?

C. The Cost of Convenience Foods—Ready-to-Eat Products, Packaged Mixes

Examine several ready-to-eat and packaged mixes of convenience foods. Compare cost per serving of convenience foods to the same product prepared from scratch (e.g., baked items, puddings, etc.).

Type of Food	Brand and Product	Cost/Serving
1. "Scratch" Form		
Packaged Mix		
Ready-to-Eat		
2. "Scratch" Form		
Packaged Mix		
Ready-to-Eat		

1. What is the relationship between convenience and price?

2. What factors may influence a consumer's choice of product form?

D. Comparing Price per Serving of Various Forms of a Food

1. Milk

Compare several milk products (as available) and complete the following chart:[a]

Form of Milk	Unit	Cost/Unit	Cost/Serving[b]	Uses of Product
Nonfat dry milk (national brand)	Bulk			
Nonfat dry milk (store brand)	Bulk			
Evaporated, whole	12 oz. (360 mL)			

Form of Milk	Unit	Cost/Unit	Cost/Serving[b]	Uses of Product
Evaporated, skim	12 oz. (360 mL)			
Fresh, whole	1 qt. (1 L)			
Fresh, 2%	1 qt. (1 L)			
Fresh, skim	1 qt. (1 L)			

[a] For laboratory purposes, use quart or liter as market unit.
[b] 8 fl. oz. (240 mL), or as reconstituted to 8 oz. (240 mL).

1. How do the form and brand of milk affect price?

2. State how "unit pricing" assists consumers in determining the best buy for the money spent.

3. Discuss how the various forms of milk could be used in order to take advantage of price differences.

2. Potatoes

Compare several potato products. Calculate cost per serving[a] and suggest possible uses.

Form of Potato	Cost/Unit	Cost/Serving	Possible Uses of Product
Idaho baker			
Potatoes (regular)			
Canned potatoes			
Dried potato flakes			
Frozen French fries			
Frozen hash browns			

[a] See Appendix C.

1. What factors influence the form of potatoes that will be chosen for dinner by an individual?

2. How will the *season* of the year affect the above price comparison?

3. How does the *geographic location* of a consumer affect the price paid for food?

E. Cost Comparison of Food, As Purchased (A.P.) and Edible Portion (E.P.)

Compare the cost per pound (454 g), as purchased (A.P.) to cost per pound (454 g), edible portion (E.P.).

Food	Cost/lb. (g) A.P.	Percent Waste[a]	Weight E.P.	Cost/lb. (g) E.P.
Apple		8		
Banana		32		
Broccoli		22		
Carrot		18–22		
Orange		25–32		
Fresh peas (in pod)		62		
Chicken, fryer		32		
Haddock, fillet		0		

[a] *Source:* Watt, B.K. and A.L. Merrill. 1963. *Composition of Foods: Raw, Processed, Prepared*. Agricultural Handbook No. 8. Washington, DC: U.S. Department of Agriculture, Consumer and Food Economics Research Division.

1. What factors influence the percentage of *waste* in a food?

2. How is information about percent waste of *value* to the consumer?

EXERCISE 2: LABELS AS GUIDES IN FOOD PURCHASING

PROCEDURE

1. Complete the table by viewing the samples of products displayed or by visiting a grocery market.
2. Share information and answers with classmates.

Product	Label Information Type

1. What product label information assists you in food purchasing decisions?

2. What government regulations and federal agency specify criteria for labeling?

3. What label format or information, not currently provided, would be useful to consumers?

4. Identify how labels may be guides in purchasing of foods for special dietary needs such as food allergies.

EXERCISE 3: "HEALTH" FOOD

Compare several versions of food products, including "health" food. Calculate cost per serving[a] and suggest possible benefits.

Food Product	Cost/Unit	Cost/Serving	Possible Benefits

EXERCISE 4: PLANNED-OVER FOODS

PROCEDURE

1. List (no prep) several foods that may be deliberately planned to yield leftovers for home or work.
2. Identify cost–benefits, microbial concerns, nutrient retention strategies, and reheating options.

Planned-Over Food	Cost–Benefit	Microbial Concerns	Nutrient Retention	Reheating Options

3. In the chart, summarize leftover food appearance, texture, and flavor for the following foods:

Food	Appearance	Texture	Flavor
Soup			
Meat			
Meat alternative			
Potato			
Rice			
Noodles			
Vegetables			
Dessert			
Other			

SUMMARY QUESTIONS—ECONOMIC DIMENSIONS

1. Summarize the diverse factors that influence prices of food.

2. Based on comparisons of various food products, list major factors a consumer might consider in selecting good money buys.

JUST THINK:

In practice, what factors, other than price, do consumers take into account when selecting food in the marketplace?

B. Nutritional Dimensions

Let food be your medicine and medicine be your food.

— **Hippocrates**

Objectives

To identify standard serving size of selected foods
To identify factors influencing caloric value of foods
To compute nutritive values of selected foods
To generalize the major nutrient contributions of groups in the Pyramid
To recognize the advantages and disadvantages of food guides
To use the Pyramid and Dietary Guidelines to evaluate a dietary plan
To recognize the major foods causing food allergies

References[1]

Appendices B, C, D, E
http://vm.cfsan.fda.gov/~lrd/cf101-12.html (standard serving size Table 2)
www.MyPyramid.gov
www.eatright.org
www.ific.org
http://www.cfsan.fda.gov
http://www.cfsan.fda.gov/label.html
www.diabetes.org
www.aicr.org
http://www.aicr.org/publications/nap/ssw.lasso (standard serving sizes for average adults)
http://www.nhlbi.nih.gov/health/public/heart/hbp/dash/nic.org/

[1] Websites current at time of printing.

http://my.clevelandclinic.org/disorders/allergies/hic_living_with_a_food_allergy.aspx
http://my.clevelandclinic.org/disorders/allergies/hic_Problem_Foods_Is_it_an_Allergy_or_Intolerance.aspx

Terms

Allergen
Dietary Guidelines
Food Guides
Functional Food
Labels
MyPyramid.gov
NRC/NAS
Nutrition Facts
RDI, RDA
Standard serving size

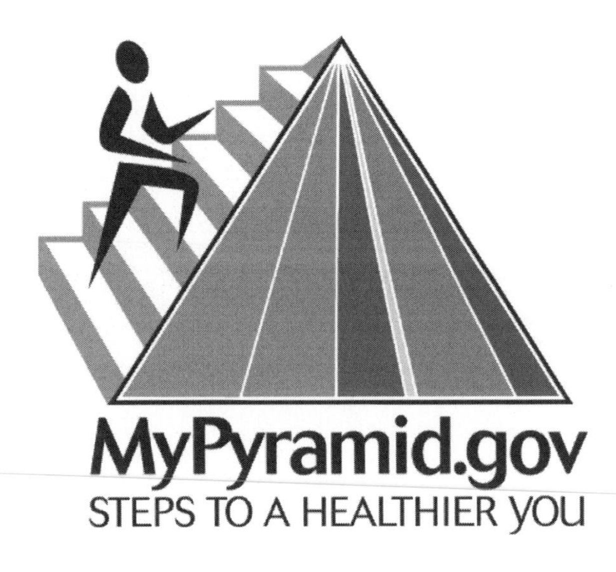

To see portion size, go to: Spotlights

- Go to Inside the Pyramid
- Go to Related Topics
- Go to View Food Gallery
- Select Food to see portions

EXERCISE 1: DETERMINING SERVING SIZE

Procedure

1. Observe a demonstration or calculate the standard serving size of several foods or food models.
2. Record weight/measure in the table.
3. Display food or food models; see pictures of portion sizes on MyPyramid.gov.
4. Compare your personal conception of a serving with the standard serving size.

Food	Standard Serving Size Weight/Measure	Comments
Bread		
Crackers		
Pasta		
Peanut butter		
Meat, poultry, fish		
Cooked legumes		
Cooked vegetables		
Canned fruits		
Whole fruits		
Ice cream		
Other		

EXERCISE 2: FACTORS AFFECTING CALORIC VALUE OF FOODS

Procedure

1. Observe a demonstration or calculate 100-calorie portions of apple products.
2. Display and compare sizes of portions. Record observations.

	Raw Apple	Applesauce	Apple Pie
100-kcal portion size			

What are some of the factors that affect the caloric value of these apple products?

EXERCISE 3: NUTRIENT CONTRIBUTIONS OF THE FOOD PYRAMID

PROCEDURE

1. Using the portion size reference listed, determine the standard serving size of foods in the group of foods assigned. (These groups do not represent a daily menu!)

A	B	C
skim milk egg frozen peas black bean soup peanut butter lettuce	whole milk canned pineapple beets pork chop canned peas corn flakes black-eyed peas process(ed) cheese	apple cheddar cheese hamburger macaroni potato, white sweet potato/yam tortilla
D	**E**	**F**
canned peaches yogurt tomato taco collard greens kidney beans rice carrots, raw	celery margarine spinach/kale orange tuna fish tomato juice bread, enriched grapes	cottage cheese biscuit fresh green beans lasagna fish fillet cabbage pancakes frosted cereal

2. Calculate and record the nutritive value of standard servings in assigned group(s) A to F, under the appropriate headings on the following chart.
3. Optional: Display servings of foods or food models, with a chart of completed nutritive value. Arrange foods on display table according to the Food Pyramid.

Nutritive Contributions of the Food Pyramid									
Food Group	Wt/Measure per Serving	Energy (kcal)	Protein (g)	Fat (g)	Carb. (g)	Vitamin A (%)	Vitamin C (%)	Calcium (%)	Iron (%)
Grains									
Vegetables									
Fruit									

Nutritive Contributions of the Food Pyramid

Food Group	Wt/Measure per Serving	Energy (kcal)	Protein (g)	Fat (g)	Carb. (g)	Vitamin A (%)	Vitamin C (%)	Calcium (%)	Iron (%)
Milk									
Meat and beans									
Fats									

EXERCISE 4: EVALUATION OF A DAILY MENU

PROCEDURE

Using the charts below, evaluate the following by the Food Pyramid.

Breakfast

Orange juice (½ cup [120 mL])
Cheese omelet (2 eggs, ½ oz. [14 g] cheese)
Whole wheat toast (2), buttered (½ tsp [2.5 mL])
Strawberry jam (2 Tbsp [30 mL])

Lunch

Navy bean soup (¼ cup [60 mL] beans)
Saltines (4)
Spinach salad (1 cup [240 mL])
Yogurt dressing (¼ cup [60 mL])
Fig bar cookie (2)

Dinner

Chicken tetrazzini (2 oz. [57 g] chicken, ½ oz. [14 g] cheese, ½ cup [120 mL] spaghetti)
Green beans (¾ cup [180 mL]), buttered (½ tsp [2.5 mL])
Carrot sticks (½ cup [120 mL])
Strawberry gelatin (½ cup [120 mL])
Milk, whole (8 oz. [240 mL])

Grains	Vegetables	Fruits

Meat and Beans	Milk	Oils

EXERCISE 5: LABELS AS GUIDES TO NUTRIENT CONTENT

PROCEDURE

1. Complete the tables by viewing samples of products displayed or by visiting a grocery.
2. Share information and answers with classmates.

A. NUTRITIVE VALUE AND COST OF FRUIT-JUICE PRODUCTS

Study the labels of several fruit-juice products (e.g., juice, punch, frozen, powdered) and compare costs and vitamin C content.

Brand and Product	Cost/Cup (240 mL)	Vitamin C/Cup (240 mL)	Fruit Juice (%)

1. Considering the vitamin C content, which is the best buy? Why?

2. Considering the percentage natural *fruit juice* content, which is the best buy?

3. What other criteria for judgment are important to you as a consumer of a juice product? Explain.

B. CARBOHYDRATE LABEL INFORMATION

PROCEDURE

Study the illustration of carbohydrate information that appears on cereal product labels.

Total carbohydrates in 1 oz. (28 g)	20 g
Dietary fiber	3 g
Sugar	5 g
Other carbohydrates	12 g

1. Specify what is meant by carbohydrate "sugars" and "other."

2. Concerning the 5 g of sugar in this 1-oz. serving, what is the measure equivalent?

3. Define "dietary fiber." How does it differ from "crude fiber"?

C. Nutritive Value and Cost of Cereal Products

Study the labels of several dry-cereal products currently on the market. Complete the following chart, selecting two cereals for comparison. (See the sample at the end of this chapter.)

	Brand 1	Brand 2
Serving size		
Servings per container		
Calories		
Calories from fat		
Total fat		
Saturated fat		
Trans fat		
Cholesterol		
Sodium		
Potassium		
Total carbohydrates		
Dietary fiber		
Sugars		
Other carbohydrates		
Protein		

1. Were all the cereal labels equally helpful in determining the nutritive value? Explain.

2. Based on the label information, which cereal is the best "nutritive" buy? Which is the "best buy" for you? Why?

3. What more does the ingredients list tell you about the specific ingredients in a product?

D. Health Claims Allowed on Labels

View health claims on food packages. Be able to specify the allowed nutrient-disease relationship claims, and rules for their use on food products, for example, fat, fiber, saturated fat, cholesterol, sodium, calcium, folate, sugar alcohols, soluble fiber, soy, whole grains, plant sterols, potassium, and so forth. Describe "functional food."

E. Food Allergies

1. Define a food allergy.

2. Define a food intolerance.

3. Identify the major food component causing allergies.

4. Based on the references, identify protein ingredients known to cause allergies.

5. Eating with food allergies impacts many dimensions of food, nutrition, and the individual's sense of well-being. Describe several recipe adjustments needed for successful preparation of food that does not contain known allergens.

6. What are allergen food labeling requirements? (See Appendix E.)

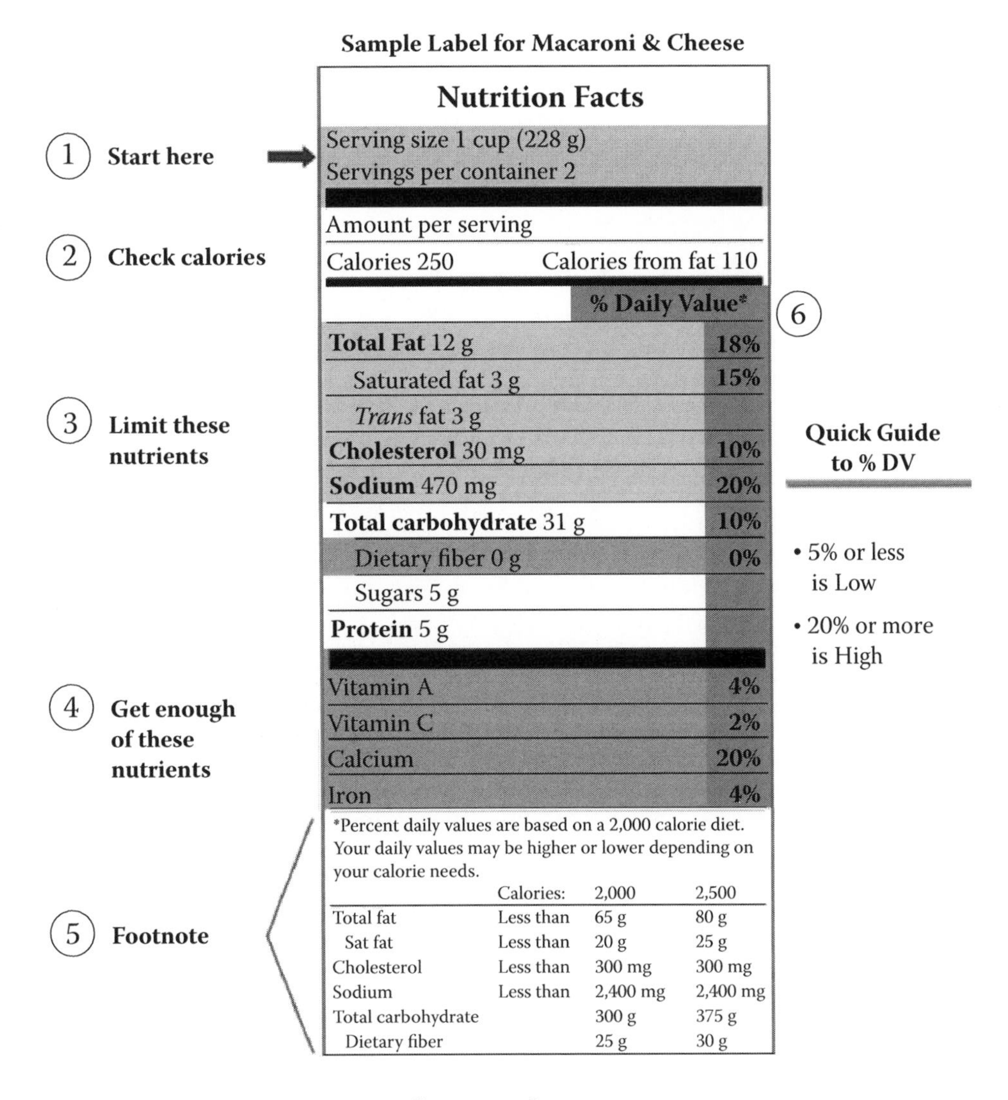

SUMMARY OF LABELING.
HTTP://WWW.CFSAN.FDA.GOV/~DMS/FOODLAB.HTML

SUMMARY QUESTIONS—NUTRITIONAL DIMENSIONS

1. Provide examples of how the caloric value of some vegetables and meats can be increased by methods of preparation.

2. Consider your own personal food preferences and habits. What individual foods in each group of the Food Pyramid act as personal safeguard foods for obtaining a regular supply of the major nutrients?

Food Group	Individual Foods
Bread	
Vegetables	
Fruit	
Meat	
Milk	

3. Of current concern are the amounts of fat and cholesterol in the American diet. List several foods that supply significant amounts of these items. List suggestions for improving the diet.

4. Consider the foods that comprise the Pyramid. What generalizations (e.g., high/low value) can be made regarding the major nutritive contributions of each food group listed?

Group	Protein	Carbohydrate	Fat	Vitamin A	Vitamin C	Iron	Calcium
Bread							
Vegetables							
Fruit							
Milk							
Meat and beans							
Fats							

5. As the director of a Head Start school, you are concerned about the feeding program available to your children, especially breakfast. Because your cook is not on duty until 9:00 a.m., some provision must be made to serve a nutritious breakfast, yet one that does not involve cooking. You are considering a new product called "Magic Muffin," which tastes like a frosted cupcake, but is highly fortified. Briefly discuss some of the aspects you will need to consider before you make a final decision.

6. Are there occasions where nutrition wins out over other considerations in choosing which food to eat? Explain.

7. a. List two advantages to the consumer of the nutrition facts/allergen labels on food products.

   b. What additional nutrition information would you like to see on labels of food products?

JUST THINK:

At what age is it appropriate to introduce good nutrition to a child?

C. Palatability Dimensions

Man is born to eat.

— **Craig Claiborne**

Objectives

To identify the major sensory properties of food
To describe sensory characteristics responsible for perception of flavor
To evaluate a product in various forms as to sensory properties and personal preferences
To identify various sensory tests used for evaluation of food acceptability
To evaluate foods marketed for use with food allergies

References

MyPyramid.gov

Assigned Readings

www.ift.org

Terms

Appearance	Flavor	Ranking Test	Tenderness
Aroma	Moistness	Sensory testing	Texture
Consistency	Mouthfeel	Subjective testing	Triangle Difference Test
Duo-Trio Difference Test	Off-flavor	Temperature	

In the following sections, exercises are presented to illustrate some factors that affect the palatability of food and food decisions. Some of the exercises may be completed independently.

EXERCISE 1: IDENTIFYING SENSORY PROPERTIES OF FOOD

PROCEDURE

1. Sample foods of each category listed on the chart.
2. Categorize the predominant sensory properties, using terms 1 through 5 in the chart below.
3. Describe sensory properties as fully as possible. Compare and contrast samples in each section of the chart. Discuss observations with classmates.

Principal Sensory Properties of Food
Appearance Texture ("mouthfeel") Flavor—taste and odor Odor or aroma Temperature

Food	Predominant Sensory Property	Description
Standard—1 cup water (240 mL)		
1 cup water + 1 tsp sugar (5 mL)		
1 cup water + 1 tbsp sugar (15 mL)		
1 cup water + 2 tsp lemon juice (10 mL)		
1 cup water + 2 tsp lemon juice (10 mL) + 1 tsp sugar (10 mL)		
1 cup water + ½ tsp salt (2.5 mL)		
1 cup water + ½ tsp salt (2.5 mL) + ½ tsp sugar (2.5 mL)		
Raw onion		
Raw apple		
Raw potato		
Cold ice cream		
Melted ice cream		
Gelatin (solid)		
Gelatin (liquid soft)		
Mineral oil		
Crackers		
Celery		
Angel food cake		
Pickles		
Mints		

(continued on next page)

Food	Predominant Sensory Property	Description
White bread		
Sample plain tomato juice. Add different seasonings singly and taste. Rinse mouth with water between samples. Compare and contrast the effect of different seasonings.		
Examples: sugar, salt, lemon juice, basil, Worcestershire sauce, tarragon, oregano		
Other:		

Grains Make half your grains whole	Vegetables Vary your veggies	Fruits Focus on fruits	Milk Get your calcium-rich foods	Meat & Beans Go lean with protein
Eat at least 3 oz. of whole-grain cereals, breads, crackers, rice, or pasta every day 1 oz. is about 1 slice of bread, about 1 cup of breakfast cereal, or ½ cup of cooked rice, cereal, or pasta	Eat more dark-green veggies like broccoli, spinach, and other dark leafy greens Eat more orange vegetables like carrots and sweetpotatoes Eat more dry beans and peas like pinto beans, kidney beans, and lentils	Eat a variety of fruit Choose fresh, frozen, canned, or dried fruit Go easy on fruit juices	Go low-fat or fat-free when you choose milk, yogurt, and other milk products If you don't or can't consume milk, choose lactose-free products or other calcium sources such as fortified foods and beverages	Choose low-fat or lean meats and poultry Bake it, broil it, or grill it Vary your protein routine — choose more fish, beans, peas, nuts, and seeds
For a 2,000-calorie diet, you need the amounts below from each food group. To find the amounts that are right for you, go to MyPyramid.gov.				
Eat 6 oz. every day	Eat 2½ cups every day	Eat 2 cups every day	Get 3 cups every day; for kids aged 2 to 8, it's 2	Eat 5½ oz. every day

Find your balance between food and physical activity

- Be sure to stay within your daily calorie needs.
- Be physically active for at least 30 minutes most days of the week.
- About 60 minutes a day of physical activity may be needed to prevent weight gain.
- For sustaining weight loss, at least 60 to 90 minutes a day of physical activity may be required.
- Children and teenagers should be physically active for 60 minutes every day, or most days.

Know the limits on fats, sugars, and salt (sodium)

- Make most of your fat sources from fish, nuts, and vegetable oils.
- Limit solid fats like butter, stick margarine, shortening, and lard, as well as foods that contain these.
- Check the Nutrition Facts label to keep saturated fats, *trans* fats, and sodium low.
- Choose food and beverages low in added sugars. Added sugars contribute calories with few, if any, nutrients.

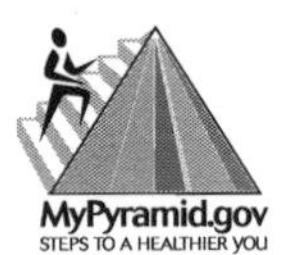

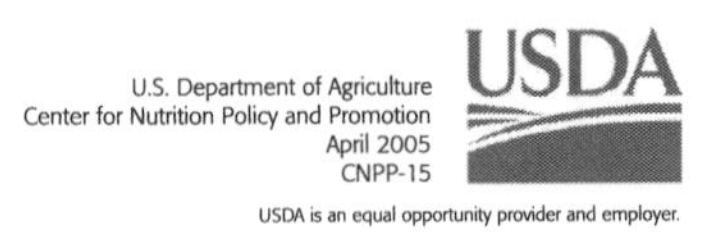

1. How does *temperature* affect perception of flavor?

2. How do basic tastes differ when used *together*?

3. For what foods is *odor* or *aroma* the predominant sensation?

4. Explain how a "standard," the cup of plain water, is helpful in evaluating sensory properties.

EXERCISE 2: SENSORY EVALUATION TESTS

PROCEDURE

1. Design an experiment using the following tests for a product[a] and/or a new ingredient in a product:
   a. **Triangle Difference Test**. A comparison of three numbered samples on a plate, including one different item out of three, to determine whether the different attribute can be detected. Circle the number of the **different** sample, or *use the ballot provided at the end of this chapter.*

      1. 2. 3.

   b. **Duo-Trio Difference Test**. A reference and two numbered samples on a plate. Circle the one that is **similar** to the reference or *use the ballot provided at the end of this chapter.*

      Reference 1. 2.

   c. **Ranking**. This test is a comparison of several food samples by ranking them according to preference. Rank samples or *use the form provided at the end of this chapter.*
2. Taste various food items, evaluating products using the assigned tests.
3. Record a critique of the test used.

Food Item	Test Used	Critique of Test Used

[a] Suggested products: beverage sweetened with aspartame/sugar, regular/light cheese, regular/low-salt or no-salt crackers.

EXERCISE 3: EVALUATING SENSORY PROPERTIES IN FOODS

PROCEDURE

1. Compare sensory properties of a single product that has been processed in different ways. *Examples:* macaroni and cheese, pudding, baked item: "scratch"/ packaged/canned/frozen.
2. Describe the blend of sensory properties characteristic of any product that was sampled.
3. State which product you preferred. Explain your choice based on personal preference and sensory properties.

Food Product	Sensory Properties (see chart above)	Preferences and Reasons
1 a.		
b.		
c.		
d.		
2 a.		
b.		
c.		
d.		

EXERCISE 4: EVALUATING FOOD PRODUCTS MARKETED FOR USE WITH FOOD ALLERGIES

PROCEDURE

1. Compare sensory properties of several products that have been processed/manufactured to accommodate food allergies (for example, lactose intolerance, gluten-free, and so forth).
2. Mark which product is preferred. Identify sensory properties and explain your choice based on personal preference.

Food Product	Sensory Properties (see chart above)	Reasons for Preference
1 a.		
b.		
2 a.		
b.		
3 a.		
b.		

EXERCISE 5: EVALUATING PERSONAL PREFERENCES

Procedure

1. Survey several classmates regarding their food preferences, using the following questionnaire format.
2. List four favorite foods, then check categories that are associated with those foods.

Favorite Foods	Family	Peers	Comfort	Celebration	Nutrition	Other

3. List four disliked foods, then check the palatability characteristics associated with those foods.

Disliked Foods	Appearance	Flavor	Texture	Other

SUMMARY QUESTIONS—PALATABILITY DIMENSIONS

1. Discuss how perception of "eating quality" may be influenced by past experiences.

2. Analyze your favorite food, identifying sensory properties and personal factors that make it your favorite.

3. Based on your survey, what are the major palatability characteristics that influence the acceptability of foods?

4. With another individual, select a food that you both like. Together, write a description of the desired properties or the standards you would expect. Do you both agree on all points? Check your description against standard descriptions (product standards in this manual or other textbooks).

JUST THINK:

One must choose chef-prepared foods in order for the food to have a good appearance, texture, and flavor. True or false? Why?

REFERENCE MATERIAL: OVERVIEW, BALLOTS, RATING

Subjective vs. Objective Analysis—Overview

Subjective/Sensory Analysis	***Objective Analysis***
Uses individuals	Uses equipment
Involves human sensory organs	Uses physical and chemical techniques
Results may vary	Results are repeatable
Determines human sensitivity to changes in ingredients, processing, or packaging	Need to find a technique appropriate for the food being tested
Determines consumer acceptance	Cannot determine consumer acceptance unless correlated with sensory testing
Time-consuming and expensive	Generally faster, cheaper, and more efficient than sensory testing
Essential for product development and for marketing of new products	Essential for routine quality control

Source: V.A. Vaclavik and E.W. Christian. 2008. ***Essentials of Food Science***, 3rd edition. New York: Springer.

TEST#_____ Panelist#_____

TRIANGLE DIFFERENCE TEST

PRODUCT_____

INSTRUCTIONS: Proceed when you are ready (quietly so as not to distract others).

FOR EACH SAMPLE:

1) Take a bite of the cracker and a sip of water to rinse your mouth.

2) Two of the samples are the same and one is different. **CIRCLE** the **ODD** sample. If you cannot tell, guess.

_____ _____ _____

3) Describe the reason why the ODD sample is DIFFERENT. (Please be specific.)

Ballot for the Triangle Sensory Test (obtained from Dr. Clay King at the Sensory Testing Laboratory at Texas Woman's University, Denton, Texas).

TEST#_____ Panelist#_____

DUO-TRIO DIFFERENCE TEST

PRODUCT_____

INSTRUCTIONS: Proceed when you are ready (quietly so as not to distract others).

FOR EACH SAMPLE:

1) Take a bite of the cracker and a sip of water to rinse your mouth.

2) **CIRCLE** the number of the sample which is **THE SAME** as the reference R. If you cannot tell, guess.

R _____ _____

3) Why are R and the sample you chose the same?

Ballot for the Duo-Trio Sensory Test (obtained from Dr. Clay King at the Sensory Testing Laboratory at Texas Woman's University, Denton, Texas).

The following was obtained from Dr. Clay King at the Sensory Testing Laboratory at Texas Woman's University, Denton, Texas.

TEST#_____ **Panelist#_____**

LIKEABILITY RATING AND PAIRED PREFERENCE TEST

PRODUCT_____

INSTRUCTIONS: Proceed when you are ready (quietly so as not to distract others). Evaluate one sample at a time, working from top to bottom.

FOR EACH SAMPLE:

1) Take a bite of the cracker and a sip of water to rinse your mouth.

2) Taste the sample then **CIRCLE** the number which best expresses your opinion of the sample.

SAMPLE CODE:_____

Likeability	1	2	3	4	5	6	7	8	9
Scale	Dislike Extremely							Like Extremely	

SAMPLE CODE:_____

Likeability	1	2	3	4	5	6	7	8	9
Scale	Dislike Extremely							Like Extremely	

Describe the DIFFERENCES between the two samples. (Please be specific.)

Taste the samples again, then circle the one you prefer.

_____ _____

Describe the reasons why you prefer the one you chose.

D. Chemical Dimensions[1]

Yuck, this stuff is full of ingredients!

— Linus, reading a can label in *Charlie Brown*

Objectives

To recognize the general role of food additives in specific foods
To identify the ingredients classified as food additives from food labels
To understand the laws regulating the use of additives
To relate the extent of processing and use of additives
To evaluate and interrelate the nutritional value, cost, and use of additives
To identify the significance of labeling on foods to show ingredients

References

Appendices E, F, G

Pennington, J.A. and J.S. Douglass. 2004. ***Bowes and Church's Food Values of Portions Commonly Used,*** 18th edition. Philadelphia, PA: Lippincott Williams & Wilkins.

Terms

Antioxidant	Food additive	Hazard	Sequestrant
Delaney Clause	Food Additive Amendment	Humectant	Stabilizer
Emulsifier	Fortification	Maturing agent	Synergist
Enrichment	GRAS	Risk	Toxicity

[1] All foods are composed of chemicals. The focus here is on nutritive and nonnutritive chemicals added to foods for specific purposes.

GRAS Ingredients in Common Foods				
Breads	Soft Drinks	Cheeses	Cake Mixes	Canned Fruits/Vegetables
Preservatives Sequestrants Surfactants Bleaching agents Nutrients	Preservatives Antioxidants Sequestrants Thickeners Acids Coloring agents Nonnutritive sweeteners Nutrients Flavoring agents	Preservatives Sequestrants Thickeners Acids Coloring agents	Antioxidants Sequestrants Surfactants Thickeners Bleaching agents Acids Coloring agents Nonnutritive sweeteners Flavoring agents	Antioxidants Thickeners Alkalis Coloring agents Nonnutritive sweeteners Thickeners Alkalis Coloring agents Nonnutritive sweeteners

Source: The Sciences, Vol. 14, No. 5, July/August, 1974. © The New York Academy of Sciences. Reprinted with permission.

EXERCISE 1: FUNCTIONS OF FOOD ADDITIVES

PROCEDURE

1. List several major functions of food additives.
2. Study the labels of the foods on display in the laboratory or visit a supermarket.
3. Identify additives that illustrate the functions listed.
4. Note also the products in which the additives are found.
5. Record all information on the following chart.

Additive Function	Specific Additive	Products Containing Additive

EXERCISE 2: RELATIONSHIP OF ADDITIVE USE TO DEGREE OF PROCESSING

PROCEDURE

1. Compare food products[2] prepared from "scratch," packaged mix, and purchased ready-to-eat (RTE).
2. Complete the following table after analyzing the ingredients used in the preparation of the various products.

Ingredients		
Prepared "from Scratch"	Packaged Mix	Ready-to-Eat

1. Summarize the relationship between degree of processing and additive use.

2. Identify reasons why one form of the product may be more beneficial to a consumer than the alternatives.

[2] Suggested products: main dish item, bakery item, pudding, and gravy.

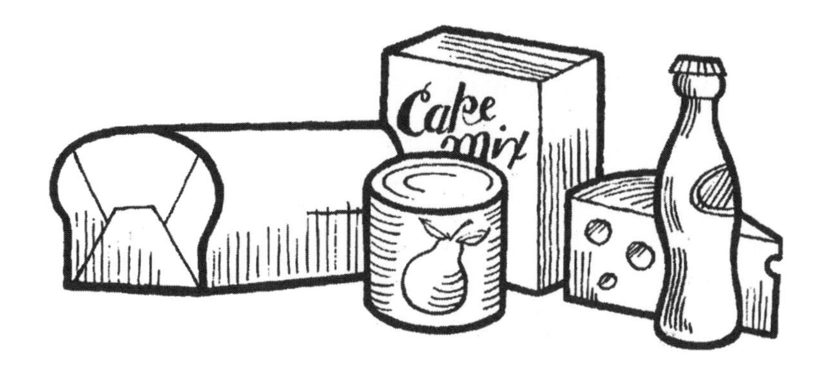

EXERCISE 3: EVALUATION OF SNACK FOODS

PROCEDURE

1. From appropriate tables calculate and complete the chart with weight and measure of 100-calorie portions of the assigned snack foods.[3]
2. If the snack foods are available, place on display and label with weight and measure. Note additives.
3. Put a star (*) next to those snacks that are high in simple sugars, and a double-star (**) next to those high in fat. Put a check (√) next to those snacks that have a high sodium content.

Snack Food Item	Weight, Measure 100-kcal portion	Major Nutrients	Additives

Conclusions:

[3] Suggestions: potato chips, pretzels, air-popped buttered popcorn, sour-cream dip, peanuts, pizza, chocolate bar, bagel, cookie, ice cream, fresh fruit, juice, carbonated drink, and so forth.

EXERCISE 4: SODIUM CONTENT OF FOODS

PROCEDURE

Using appropriate references, complete the following chart on the sodium content of common foods.

Food Item	Measure	Sodium Content (mg)	No/Low-Sodium Food (mg)
Tomato, fresh	1 medium		
Canned	1 cup (240 mL)		
Soup	1 cup (240 mL)		
Ketchup	1 tbsp (15 mL)		
Potato, baked	1 medium		
Packaged	½ cup (120 mL)		
Dairy Milk	1 cup (240 mL)		
Meat Beef, ground	3 oz. (85 g)		
Chicken	3 oz. (85 g)		
Hot dog	1		
Lunch meat	1 slice		
Bread	1 slice		
Popcorn	1 serving		
Crackers	1 serving		
Cucumber	½ large		
Dill pickle	½ large		
Soy sauce	1 tbsp (15 mL)		

1. What is the daily milligram intake of sodium suggested by dietary goals?

2. How many milligrams of sodium are there in 1 teaspoon of salt?

3. List several low-sodium and no-sodium processed foods that are available in the marketplace.

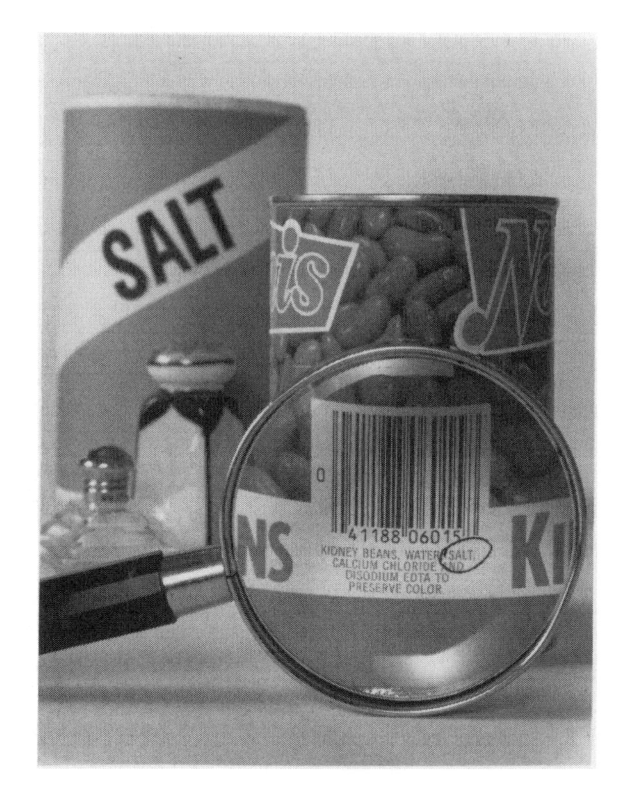

HIDDEN SALT.
Source: Division of Nutritional Sciences, New York State College of Human Ecology at Cornell University, Ithaca, NY.

EXERCISE 5: WHEAT IN FOODS

PROCEDURE

Using appropriate references, identify foods other than baked goods and cereals that contain wheat. What are some reasons for sometimes adding wheat to foods?

Food Item	Wheat Purpose

1. What foods did you not expect to contain wheat?

2. What names other than "wheat" may be on food labels?

SUMMARY QUESTIONS—CHEMICAL DIMENSIONS

1. Are all ingredients listed on a label classified as *chemicals*? Explain.

2. Are all ingredients listed on a label classified as *additives*? Explain.

3. What government regulation governs the listing of additives?

4. Provide examples of major additive functions and illustrate each with specific examples.

5. Under what circumstances are additives removed from the GRAS list?

6. Based on laboratory evaluation of snack food, what are the major nutrients in most snack food? What are the inadequacies of snack food?

7. Based on a comparison of ingredient lists on labels, what general observations can be made concerning factors that influence the number of additives used in a food?

8. Discuss the choices that a consumer has regarding the number of food additives consumed.

9. Discuss the usefulness or ease of understanding of label information for consumers who have food intolerances or food allergies.

JUST THINK:

Can I, should I, choose a diet without additives?

E. Sanitary Dimensions

Your food is close to your stomach, but you must put it in your mouth first.

— **West African saying**

Objectives

To identify factors influencing growth of microorganisms
To relate the environmental needs of bacteria
To describe the phases in the growth of bacteria
To relate key principles for evaluating sanitary quality of food
To recognize the interrelationship of the nature of food, sources of contamination, and time-temperature history of food to its sanitary quality
To describe proper sanitation of food-preparation equipment
To relate food safety to allergen-free foods

References[1]

Appendices E, H-I, H-II
http://www.ific.org/about/index.cfm
http://www.cfsan.fda.gov
Local Environmental Health Code

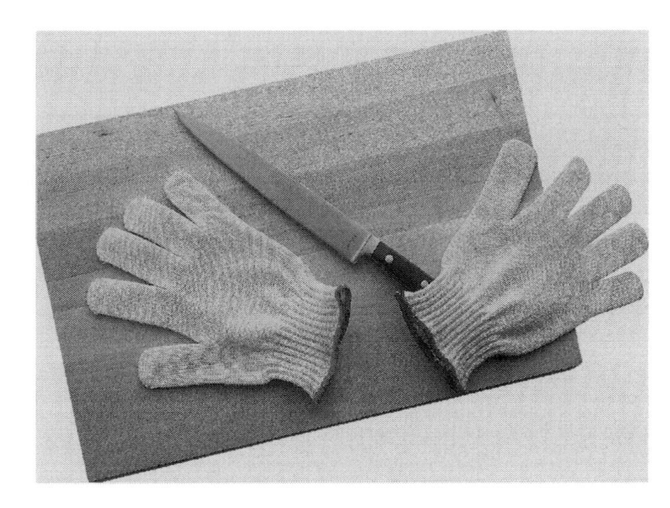

Meat-Cutting Tools.
Courtesy: SYSCO® Incorporated.

[1] Websites current at time of printing.

Terms

Aerobic
Allergen-free
Anaerobic
Bacillus cereus
Bacterial growth curve
Clostridium botulinum
Clostridium perfringens
Contaminated
Cross-contamination
FDA Model ordinance
Foodborne illness
Fungi
Infection
Intoxication
Potentially hazardous food
Salmonella sp.
Sanitization
Shigella
Spoiled
Spore
Staphylococcus aureus
Temperature danger zone
Time-temperature history
Toxin
Virus
Wholesomeness

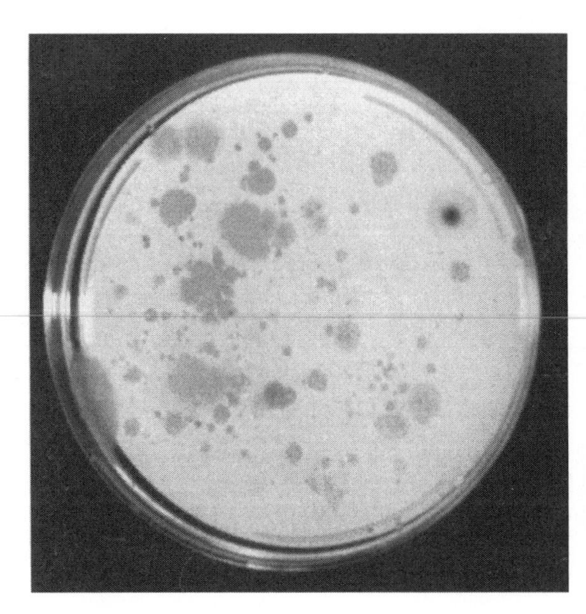

Bacterial Growth from Contaminated Apron.

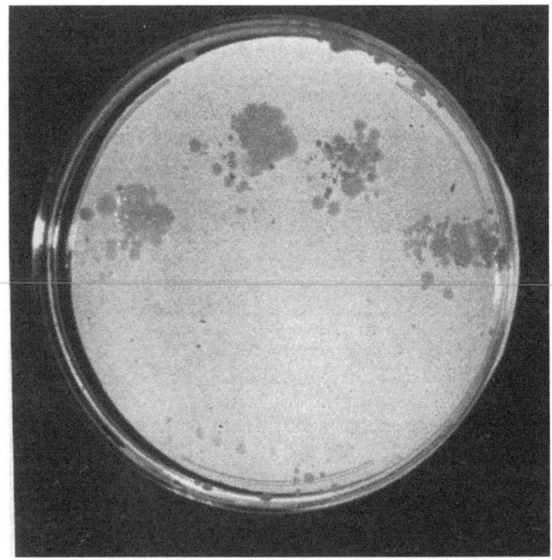

Bacterial Growth from Unwashed Hands.

Courtesy: University of Georgia, College of Agriculture.

EXERCISE 1: FACTORS AFFECTING THE MICROBIAL SAFETY OF FOODS

A. Sources of Contamination

Procedure

1. Based on readings, list common sources of food product contamination.
2. Identify methods by which contamination may be introduced into foods.

Sources of Contamination	Methods of Food Contamination

B. Conditions Necessary for the Growth of Bacteria

Procedure

1. Identify environmental conditions that bacteria need in order to grow (e.g., food, etc.).

Environmental Conditions Necessary for Bacterial Growth
a. Food—specify:
b.
c.
d.
e.
f.

2. List examples of foods that support microbial growth ("potentially hazardous foods").

C. Bacterial Growth Curve

Contaminated foods kept at unsafe temperatures, for example, 41°F to 140°F (5°C to 60°C) in the temperature danger zone become unsafe to eat after a period of time.

Procedure

1. Study the theoretical growth curve of bacteria.
2. Using references, identify what is occurring during each phase of bacterial growth.

Phase Name and Description

(a) A–B: LAG

(b) C–D: LOG

(c) E–F: STATIONARY

(d) G–H: DECLINE

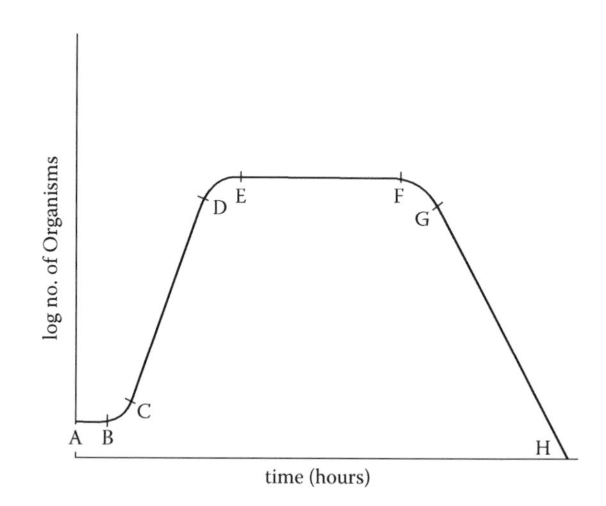

Growth Curve of Microorganisms.
Source: Frazier W.C., 1967. *Food Microbiology*. New York: McGraw-Hill. Reprinted with permission.

1. Why is there a lag in growth before numbers of bacteria begin to increase?

2. What would be the effect of refrigerating a food during the lag phase? Does freezing kill microorganisms?

3. How is microbial growth affected if a refrigerated "potentially hazardous food" were again held at room temperature, this time for several hours?

4. Explain why it is important to know the time-temperature history of foods that are to be served.

5. Summarize the conditions that must exist if an illness is to result from the ingestion of a food.

6. Explain practical control measures that should be employed to prevent foodborne illnesses.

EXERCISE 2: TEMPERATURE CONTROL IN FOOD HANDLING

A. Factors Affecting the Rate of Cooling of Large Quantities of Foods

Procedure

1. Prepare 4 qt. (or 4 L) of a boiling, thickened liquid mixture.[1]
2. Divide the liquid into four containers, using two oblong pans and two tall 1-qt. (1-L) glass measures. Record the initial temperature of the product.
3. Place one of each size container in a 40°F (4.4°C) refrigeration unit, and let the other two containers cool at room temperature.
4. Record temperatures at designated times.

[1] For laboratory purposes, use a quart or liter glass measuring cup.

Cooling Method	Temperature			
	Initial	10 min	20 min	30 min
Cooled at room temperature				
a. 1 qt. (L) measure				
b. Oblong, shallow pan				
Cooled under refrigeration				
a. 1 qt. (L) measure				
b. Oblong, shallow pan				

1. How does the ***speed*** of cooling a hot food affect the sanitary quality of that food?

2. How does the ***density or viscosity*** of the food material affect the rate of cooling?

3. In order to ensure rapid cooling and proper storage of perishable foods, what temperature range is recommended for refrigeration?

B. Temperatures for Holding and Reheating Foods

Procedure

1. Complete the chart, listing temperatures required for cold and hot holding and reheating of "potentially hazardous foods" (this may vary by state, county, or city jurisdiction).
2. Record temperature requirements for reheating of potentially hazardous foods.

	Temperature
Cold holding	
Hot holding	
Reheating	

3. Note any exceptions to these temperatures.

C. Recommended Temperatures for Cooked Food

Procedure

1. Complete the chart or take actual temperatures (see Food Safety Information at the end of this chapter regarding recommended final cooking temperatures to ensure food wholesomeness).
2. List the rationale for the temperature requirements of products.

Food Product	Temperature	Rationale for Temperature Requirements
Eggs		
Ground beef		
Pork		
Poultry		
Roast beef		
Steak		

Exercise 3: Sanitization in the Food Preparation Environment

A. Use of Approved Chemical Sanitizers

Procedure

1. Identify three chemical sanitizing agents approved by the U.S. Environmental Protection Agency for use on food contact surfaces.
2. Record concentrations of sanitizers (parts per million) required for sanitizing equipment and utensils by immersion (in a sink), and for sanitizing equipment in-place (equipment that is too large to fit in a sink, or that is electrically based and must be cleaned and sanitized in place).

Chemical Name	Concentration: Immersion	Concentration: In-Place Equipment
1. Chlorine		
2. Iodine		
3. Quaternary ammonia		
4. Other: specify		

B. Sanitization by Immersion

Procedure

1. Identify the correct arrangement of a three-compartment sink and the function of each sink compartment.

Arrangement in a Commercial/Institutional Sink	Function
First compartment sink:	
Second compartment sink:	
Third compartment sink:	

2. Specify, in the table below, the two sanitizing methods that are effective in the sanitizing sink.

Sanitizing Method	Length of Exposure Time	Water Temperature
1. Hot water		
2. Chemical		

SUMMARY QUESTIONS—SANITARY DIMENSIONS

1. Differentiate between *spoiled* and *contaminated* food products. Provide examples.

2. Why is it possible for a food to be unwholesome but not spoiled? May signs of spoilage also be indications of unwholesomeness?

3. Describe legal protection that consumers have against consuming unwholesome food.

4. Define foodborne illness. Discuss additional, emerging pathogens, not listed in Appendix G, that need to be controlled in order to prevent foodborne illness.

5. Define and distinguish between intoxication and infection.

6. Define and then explain cross-contamination using an example.

7. While commercially prepared mayonnaise (pH 3.0 to 4.1) is not a potentially hazardous food, mayonnaise-based salads (e.g., potato salad or tuna salad) are often causes of foodborne illness. Explain. Specify what ingredients, cooking procedures, and environmental factors make such foods potentially unwholesome.

8. If you, or others, associate your illness with food, to whom should the incident be reported?

9. According to the Centers for Disease Control and Prevention (CDC), roast beef and poultry are frequently reported in foodborne illness cases.
   a. Explain why this is true. Consider cooking and holding temperatures and the composition of the food.

   b. Which microorganisms are most frequently the cause of illness?

10. The following information is adapted from a case history in the Center for Disease Control.

> On March 10, 64 cases of acute gastrointestinal illness occurred among 107 guests shortly after eating at a wedding reception. The reception food was prepared in private homes and then brought to the reception. Specifically, 40 chickens were cooked and deboned on March 8, then refrigerated overnight. On March 9, the meat was ground in a meat grinder with celery and onions. Then, the mixture was mixed with mayonnaise and refrigerated. On the day of the reception (March 10), the salad was not refrigerated en route to the reception or during the reception.

Comment on this case, noting specific problems connected with the procedures that could be expected to cause illness of guests.

11. List the major factors or situations that must be studied to determine the causes of any foodborne illness. (See Exercise 1B.) Be specific in your answer.

12. A fictitious news article reads as follows:

> **75 CHILDREN ILL FROM PICNIC FOOD**
>
> SANDY POINT, U.S.A. — Poisonous food transformed a gala school picnic into mass misery Saturday night. About 75 children from Sandy Point Central School fell violently ill at their annual end-of-school picnic. Children fell ill about 3 hours after eating a delicious picnic supper.

What kind of illness would you suspect?

What foods might be involved?

Why is a picnic food often the cause of illness?

13. Identify the "Safe Handling Instructions" that appear on packaged meat and poultry. What is the reason for conveying this information to consumers?

14. Identify how the term *allergen-free* relates to food safety.

National Food Safety Education Month[SM]

Food Safety Training for Retail Food Establishments
"Cook it Safely - It's a Matter of Degrees"
Training Session

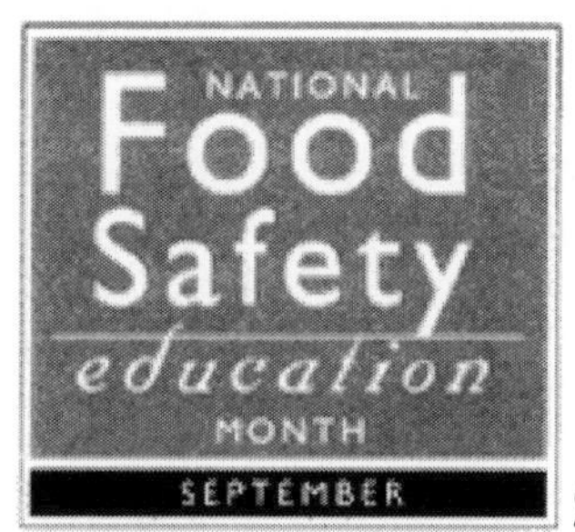

SM

Calibrating Thermometers and Taking Temperatures Properly

Part 1: Calibrating Thermometers

In this activity, you will discuss why thermometers need to be calibrated, how often they should be calibrated, and how to calibrate them. Employees will demonstrate how to correctly calibrate a thermometer of their choice.

Begin discussion by explaining that thermometers must be calibrated regularly to ensure that product temperatures are correct.

- If thermometers are used on a continual basis, they should be calibrated at least once a day. They should also be calibrated whenever the thermometer is dropped, before it is first used, and when going from one temperature extreme to another.
- There are two methods for calibrating thermometers: the ice point method and the boiling point method. Explain the steps for each method, then have employees calibrate their thermometers using either method (note to remember: the ice point method is more accurate and easier to do).

Ice Point Method:

- Fill a large glass with crushed ice. Add clean tap water until the glass is full and stir well.
- Put the thermometer stem or probe in the ice water mixture so that the entire sensing area is submerged. Do not let the stem of the thermometer or probe touch the sides or bottom of the glass. Wait at least 30 seconds or until indicator stops moving.
- With the stem of the thermometer or probe still in the ice water mixture, use a wrench to turn the adjusting nut until the thermometer reads 32°F (0°C). If calibrating a digital thermometer, press the reset button to automatically calibrate the thermometer.

Boiling Point Method:

- Bring clean tap water to a boil in a deep pan.
- Put the thermometer stem or probe into the boiling water so that the sensing area is completely submerged. Do not let the stem or probe touch the bottom or sides of the pan. Wait at least 30 seconds or until indicator stops moving.
- With the thermometer stem or probe still in the water, use a wrench to turn the adjusting nut until the thermometer reads 212°F (100°C) at sea level. If calibrating a digital thermometer, press the reset button to automatically calibrate the thermometer.

POINT TO REMEMBER:

The boiling point of water **decreases** as elevation **increases**:

Altitude (Elevation above Sea Level)	Water Boiling Point
• 0 (sea level)	• 212°F (100°C)
• 1000 feet (305 meters)	• 210°F (98.9°C)
• 2000 feet (610 meters)	• 208°F (97.8°C)
• 3000 feet (914 meters)	• 206.4°F (96.9°C)
• 4000 feet (1219 meters)	• 204.5°F (95.8°C)
• 5000 feet (1524 meters)	• 202.75°F (94.9°C)
• 8000 feet (2438 meters)	• 197.5°F (91.9°C)

Part 2: Taking Product Temperatures

In this activity, you will review how to take the temperature of various hot food items. Then, quiz your employees on how to take the temperature of various food items.

- Begin discussion by reminding employees to properly wash and sanitize their thermometers prior to use and in between uses. Also, remind employees to use the right thermometer for the food and situation, and to calibrate the thermometer whenever necessary. Key points you may want to discuss before you begin:
  - Take the temperature of a product in several places, particularly irregularly shaped items.
  - Stir product before taking temperature.
  - Place stem or probe in the thickest part of the food item.
  - Do not rest the stem or probe on a bone—this may give an inaccurate reading.
  - Make sure entire sensing area is completely submerged in the food.
  - Prior to starting this activity, set out different types of foods to have employees demonstrate how they would take the temperature of each (pretending or simply discussing can be just as useful).
- Ask employees how they would take the temperature of such food items as roast chicken, pork chops, bone-in ham, hamburgers, soup in a large stock pot on the burner, a 10 lb. roast in a large pan, or a thin sauce in a crepe pan.
- For added benefit, ask the employees what the final minimum internal temperature should be for each food item.

COMMON MISTAKES TO AVOID WHEN USING A THERMOMETER:

- Not calibrating thermometer
- Not immersing entire sensing area into product
- Taking temperature in incorrect location in the food product
- Failing to stir product prior to taking temperature
- Not using the appropriate thermometer for the type of food
- Touching the surface of the cooking vessel or equipment
- Equating air temperature with product temperature
- Equating equipment thermostat temperature with product temperature
- Failing to allow thermometer to level off
- Failing to wash and sanitize thermometer prior to use

Source: *ServSafe® Coursebook*, Chapter 5, "How to Calibrate Thermometers," pp. 5–22. Copyright 1999 The Educational Foundation of the National Restaurant Association. http://www.foodsafety.gov/~dms/sept/99-week3.html.

JUST THINK:

Identify special microbial concerns regarding use of leftovers as "planned-overs."
Practice calibrating a thermometer.

F. Food-Processing Dimensions

An expert is like the bottom of a double boiler. It shoots off a lot of steam, but it never really knows what's cooking!

— **Anonymous**

Objectives

To recognize temperatures commonly used in food processing
To identify how processing temperatures are influenced by type of processing equipment
To distinguish characteristics of standard equipment and processes used in canning and freezing
To use, compare, and evaluate common methods of canning acid and nonacid foods
To use, compare, and evaluate common methods of freezing fruits and vegetables

References

Appendiices G, H, I; USDA Cooperative Extension

Terms

Acid	Flat sour	Petcock	Simmer
Blanch	Freezer storage life	pH	Spore
Boil	Head space	Pressure canner	Syrup pack
Clostridium botulinum	Hermetic seal	Pressure cook	Toxin
Cold pack	Hot pack	Pressure sauce pan	USDA
Dry sugar pack	Low acid	Scald	Venting, exhausting
Enzymatic browning	Open kettle	Shelf life	Water bath

EXERCISE 1: PROCESSING TEMPERATURES

PROCEDURE

1. Place 2 cups (480 mL) of water in each container listed below.
2. Cover containers with lids and regulate heat to maintain temperature.
3. After 10 minutes, check and record the temperature of the water bath.

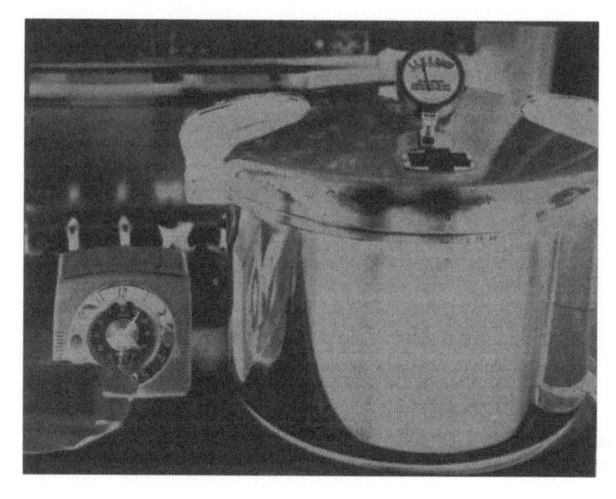

PRESSURE COOKER.
Courtesy: USDA.

Container	Temperature after 10 min
Covered saucepan (water boiling)	
Steamer	
Water in top of double boiler (over simmering water)	
Water in top of double boiler (over boiling water)	
Water in top of double boiler (surrounded by boiling water)	
Pressure saucepan (demo) (15 lb. pressure)	

1. Account for the differences in final temperature:
   a. Covered saucepan or steamer and pressure cooker at 15 lb. pressure

   b. Top of double boiler, surrounded by boiling water; top of double boiler, over boiling water

2. At what temperature does water “simmer”? Describe the appearance of the water.

3. Explain what happens when water boils. Describe the appearance of the water.

4. Compare the temperature of boiling water and the temperature of steam.

5. When will water boil at temperatures above 212°F (100°C)? Why?

6. When will water boil below 212°F (100°C)? Why?

7. How does pan shape and use of lid influence the rate of water evaporation during cooking?

8. Discuss the rate of heat transfer by conduction, convection, and radiation. Give an example of each method as used in food preparation.

EXERCISE 2: FOOD PROCESSING, CANNING

A. Canning Equipment

Procedure

1. Examine the different kinds of jars and closures available for canning. Note how closures attach to jars.
2. Examine the following processing equipment and note characteristics:
   a. Pressure canner
   b. Boiling-water bath
   c. Open kettle

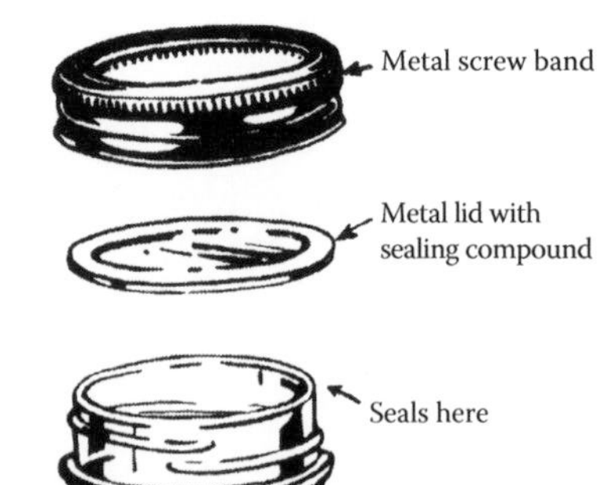

One Type of Canning Jar.
Courtesy: USDA.

B. Canning Acid and Low-Acid Foods

Procedure

1. Prepare and process 1 pint (480 mL) of vegetable (low acid) or 1 pint (480 mL) of fruit (acid). Follow current directions provided by the USDA.
2. When cool enough to handle, label the jar with the processing method used, name, and date.
3. In a subsequent laboratory, examine and evaluate canned products as to color, texture, and flavor. Complete the table below and summarize your conclusions.

Product	Relative Acidity	Canning Method	Processing		Palatability		
			Time	Temp	Color	Texture	Flavor

Conclusions:

QUESTIONS—CANNING

1. Why is the allowance of a "head space" important in packing jars for canning?

2. What foods are able to be canned in an open saucepan? What are the restrictions of using this method? Why must low-acid foods be canned in a pressure canner?

3. Must jars be sterilized when the boiling-water bath or pressure cooker is used? Explain.

4. In using the pressure canner:
   a. How and why is the canner exhausted?

   b. When is the processing time counted?

   c. Why must the pressure return to zero prior to opening the petcock and removing the cover?

5. In using the water-bath method:
   a. What temperature should the water bath be when jars are put into the bath? Why?

   b. What is the height of water in the pan, relative to the jars? Why is this important?

   c. How is "processing time" counted?

6. How are processed jars tested for a complete seal?

7. Why are screw bands removed after jars are cold and sealed?

8. Why are up-to-date references on canning essential?

9. Why does the term "processed food" sometimes carry a negative image?

EXERCISE 3: FOOD PROCESSING, FREEZING

A. Freezing Equipment

Procedure

Examine the various kinds of rigid and nonrigid freezing containers available, for example, glass jars, plastic boxes, waxed cardboard, bags, and sheets of moisture-resistant cellophane, foil, polyethylene, and so forth.

B. Freezing Fruits and Vegetables

Procedure

1. Freeze 1 pint (480 mL) of assigned fruit or vegetable, following current directions provided by the USDA, except for pretreatment indicated on the chart below.
2. Label containers and freeze.
3. In a subsequent laboratory, examine and evaluate all products. Summarize your conclusions.

Product	Pretreatment	Type of Container	Evaluation of Thawed Product
Fruit	Packed in syrup, no ascorbic acid		
Fruit	Packed in syrup, ascorbic acid		
Fruit	Dry sugar pack, ascorbic acid		
Vegetable	Blanched		
Vegetable	Unblanched		

Conclusions:

QUESTIONS—FREEZING

1. What is the function of ascorbic acid when it is added to syrup for fruits? Which fruits need ascorbic acid to ensure a palatable product?

2. Explain the role of blanching in freezing foods.

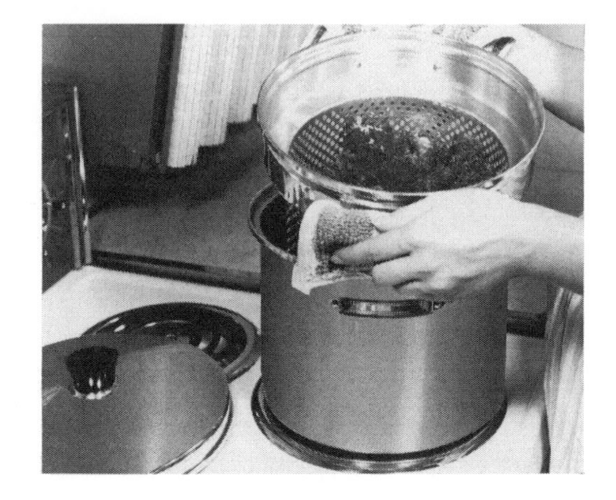

BLANCHING VEGETABLES PRIOR TO FREEZING.
Courtesy: USDA.

3. Why are vegetables chilled immediately after blanching?

4. Why must head space be allowed in freezer containers?

5. What freezer temperature is recommended for freezing and storing frozen foods?

6. How long will frozen fruits and vegetables maintain high palatability characteristics in the freezer?

7. Does freezing kill *Clostridium botulinum* spores? Explain.

8. What foods generally freeze well? What foods do not?

9. What guidelines can be used to evaluate the wholesomeness of a frozen food?

SUMMARY QUESTIONS—DIMENSIONS OF FOOD (PART I, A–F)

1. Many say variety in food choices is a basic key to good ***nutrition***. Do you agree? Why or why not?

2. You are an action worker in South America working with adolescent girls. You hear that an American company has developed Fe-ol, a new, carbonated, iron-enriched beverage. Based on the criteria for food selection, list several specific factors that you would consider and investigate before recommending that Fe-ol be used in your program.

3. With rising ***prices***, many consumers are changing food-buying habits. Discuss some ways that money can be saved on food purchased without compromising nutritive value or personal preferences.

4. As a *nutritionist* working in an underdeveloped country, you have surveyed the diets of the population and concluded that the people there were not meeting their RDAs for vitamin A, calcium, and iron. This lack was especially true for women under age 50 and for children. Your challenge is to devise and implement a basic food guide that will help improve the nutritional status of the population. After studying the food supply and dietary customs, you ascertain the following facts:
   - Most people are already eating ample quantities of rice, coffee, starchy vegetables (plantains, green bananas), lard, sugar, dried imported codfish.
   - Imported canned fruits are considered prestige foods.
   - Native citrus fruits are plentiful but are not considered prestige foods.
   - Deep-yellow fruits (papaya, mango) and vegetables (squash, sweet potato) are plentiful.
   - Dried beans can be imported at a reasonable price.
   - Eggs are fairly plentiful, often produced at home.
   - Although an island nation, fish, other than dried cod, is not plentiful.
   - Meat is high priced because it must be imported.
   - Because of a lack of refrigeration, some areas of the island do not have access to fresh milk.

Briefly discuss how you would devise an appropriate food guide. Give reasons for your choices of food groups.

5. Indicate on the thermometer the temperatures for the following situations:
   a. Temperature at which water freezes
   b. Optimum refrigerator temperature
   c. Optimum freezer temperature
   d. Temperature of simmering water
   e. Temperature of food cooking in the top of a double boiler held over simmering water
   f. Temperature of food cooking in the top of a double boiler held over boiling water
   g. Cooking at 15 lb. pressure
   h. *Salmonella* destroyed
   i. *Staphylococcus* destroyed
   j. *Clostridium perfringens* destroyed
   k. *C. botulinum* destroyed
   l. Toxin of *C. botulinum* destroyed
   m. Toxin of *Staphylococcus* destroyed
   n. Temperature for canning low-acid foods
   o. Temperature for canning acid foods

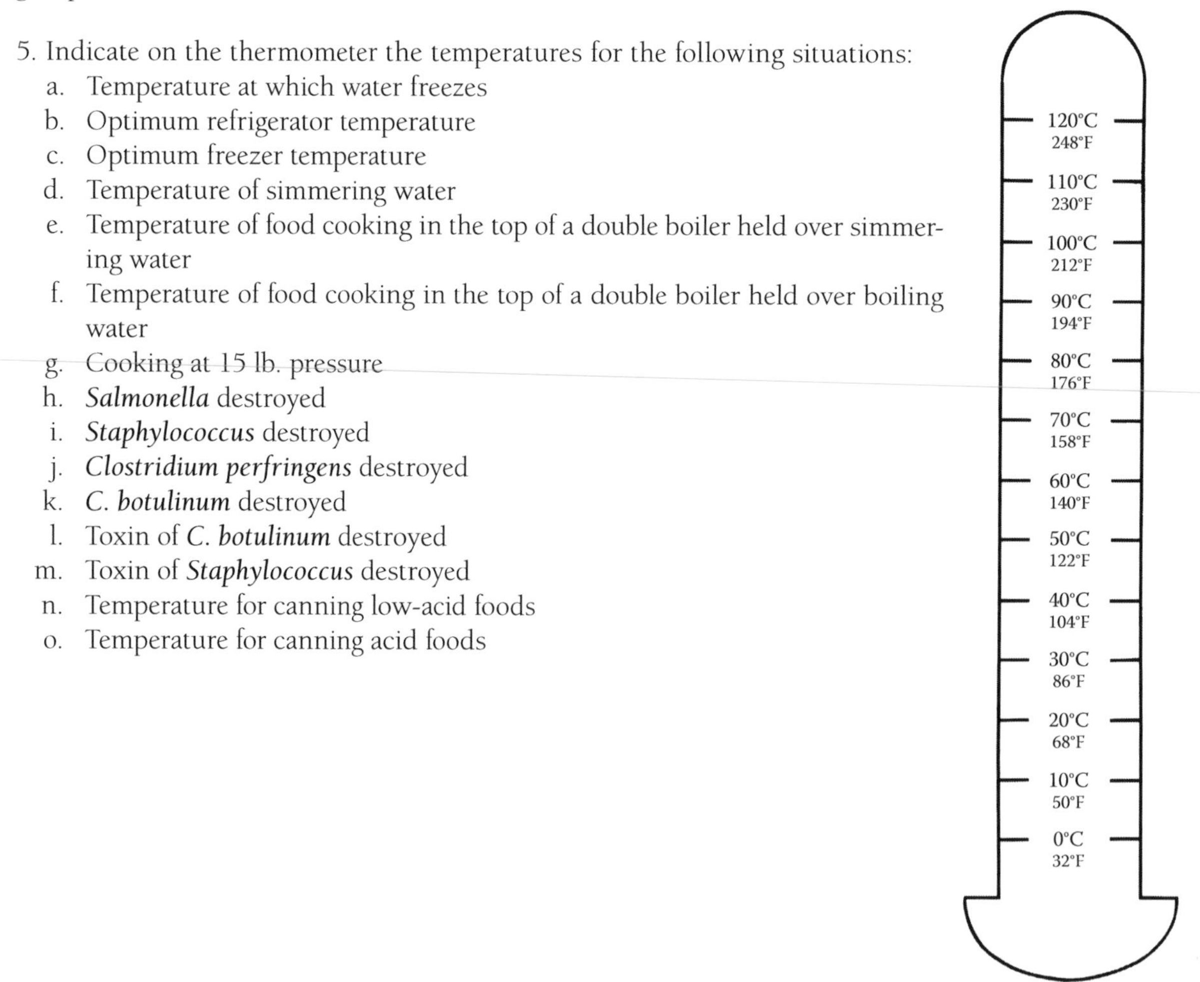

6. Bracket temperature zone of most rapid growth of microorganisms.

7. Bracket temperature zones that prevent rapid growth of microorganisms but allow their survival.

8. Keep an accurate log of all the foods you consume on a weekend. From this log, identify snacks and evaluate their ***nutritive value***.
   a. How many calories did your snacks add to your daily intake?

   b. Did any of the snacks add important nutrients you needed to meet your RDA?

9. ***Create*** a checklist to use in evaluating the ***sanitation*** practices of a restaurant or lunch counter. ***Visit*** an eating place, especially one in which you, the customer, are able to observe kitchen activities and test the validity of your checklist. Based on your observations, if you were the manager, what specific suggestions would you make to your staff concerning improved handling of foods?

10. Describe other packaging techniques such as vacuum packaging techniques that are available to the consumer at home.

11. If you have allergies, keep an accurate log of all the food allergens you could unsuspectingly consume with your typical weekend eating habits.

12. Based on your study of the *economic dimensions* of food, what suggestions would you make to food companies or to the government, for improvements that would enable shoppers to make better buys?

JUST THINK:

Why are directions for processing foods sometimes revised? What general advice would you give to anyone who plans to home-process food?

How does an individual consumer demonstrate consideration for economic, nutritional, palatability, sanitary, and processing dimensions of food and its selection?

PART II

Food Principles

Perhaps when the topic of cooking arises, you would say you *love* to cook; and that you find "success" in the kitchen! Or on the other hand, perhaps what you are making for dinner is "*reservations*"! You may believe that dining out is your best or only choice. Maybe you look at what you attempted to create in the kitchen and sarcastically say, "I'm sure *everyone* will want *that*! I totally messed up, so no cooking for me!" However, in this lab, although it might take some effort, you *can* do it!

In this manual, the functional and structural properties of food constituents and their behavior in food preparation are emphasized. Basic principles are demonstrated in a series of experiments and then applied to the preparation of various food products. Experiences with all major food groups are included. Nutritional value of these foods is emphasized, with a consideration for food allergens. Appearing as a closure to chapters is *Dietitian's Note,* which offers additional nutritional information.

Through questions and problems, your understanding of the dimensions of food, Part I, can be applied to specific food groups in Part II. From the overall experiences in this section, you will learn and be able to predict how preparation affects and changes food, not only in terms of palatability, but also in nutritive value, sanitary quality, and so forth.

Application of the principles of food preparation enhances eating, and maximizes nutritional value. This section on food principles is designed to help you understand and apply these principles.

Let's get started!

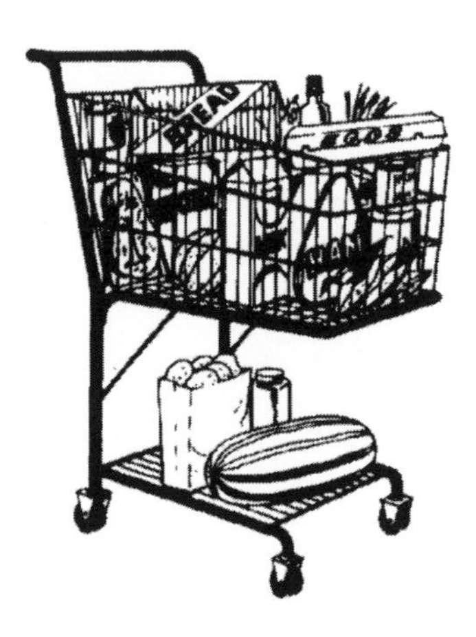

A. Measurements, Use of Ingredients, Laboratory Techniques, Policies, and Procedures

Recipes are traditions, not just random wads of ingredients.

— **Anonymous**

Objectives

To become familiar with common techniques of food preparation and cleanup
To delineate utensils and methods for measuring liquids and solids
To measure liquids and solids accurately
To recognize portion size
To become familiar with metric equivalents

References

Appendices E, J, L

Assigned Readings

Review Lab Policies and Procedures and other pertinent lab information

Terms

Beat
Chop
Dice
Fluid ounces
Fold
Meniscus
Metric equivalent
Mince
Pare
Sift
Stir

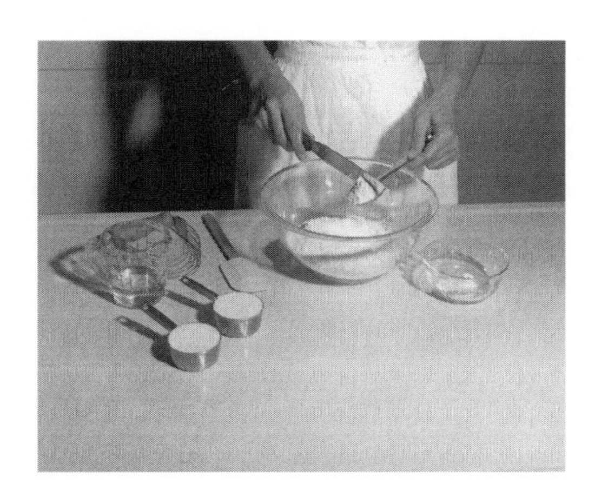

Measuring Accurately.
Source: Division of Nutritional Sciences, New York State College of Human Ecology at Cornell, Ithaca, New York.

INTRODUCTORY LABORATORY NOTES

Use of Salt and Fat

Seasoning: Salt is not included in recipes, except for yeast bread. Season to taste and limit added salt. **Use of herbs and spices is encouraged.** See Appendix N.

Use of fat: For margarine, select highly polyunsaturated brands. For oils, polyunsaturated or monounsaturated brands are suggested. Use of nonstick cooking sprays is suggested in place of greasing pans or casseroles.

Use of Milk Products

Nonfat dry milk is readily stored and may be used in recipes. To reconstitute: use ⅓ cup powder, with water added UP TO the one-cup level on a measuring cup. This yields one cup of milk. Adapt accordingly.

Use of Allergens

Please see Appendix E to note the eight major food allergens—90% of food allergens. In the preparation of food products using this manual, **not all allergens are noted in recipes**. Each student should consult with his or her doctor, and exercise caution to avoid the consumption of a known allergen.

Microwave

Refer to the chapter on Microwave Cooking for microwave oven recipes and to Appendix H for general information on heat transfer.

Environmental Consideration

You and/or your instructor may observe reuse and recycling practices that are in line with demonstrating consideration for the environment.

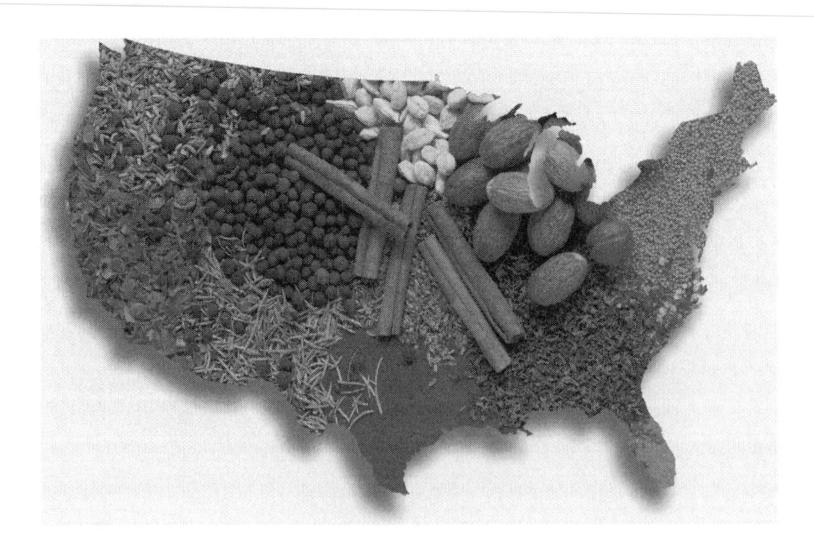

Spices in the USA.

Courtesy: SYSCO® Incorporated.

EXERCISE 1: DEMONSTRATION OF MEASURING AND MIXING TECHNIQUES

PROCEDURE

1. Observe a demonstration of measuring techniques, noting equipment for dry and liquid measures.
2. Calculate values and complete the following chart:

1 cup liquid measure	=	fluid ounces milliliters (mL) liters
1 cup dry measure	=	tablespoons (tbsp)
1 tbsp	=	teaspoons (tsp) mL
1 tsp	=	mL
1 lb. all-purpose flour	=	cups (c)
		g
1 lb. granulated sugar	=	c
		g
1 lb. butter/margarine/ shortening	=	c tbsp g
4 oz. cheddar cheese	=	g
3 oz. hamburger	=	g
3 oz. refried beans	=	g
Other:		
Other:		
Other:		

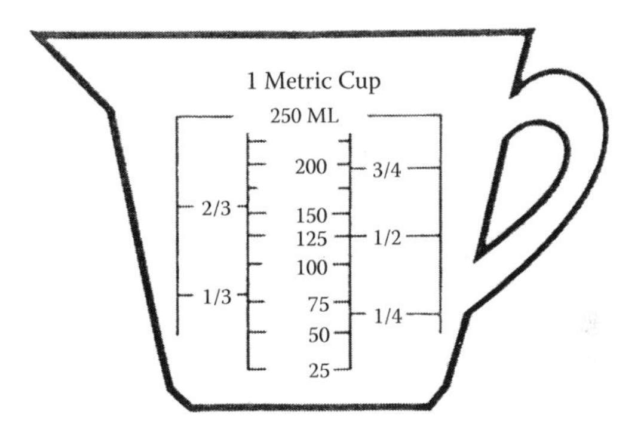

METRIC CUP.

Source: Division of Nutritional Sciences, New York State College of Human Ecology at Cornell, Ithaca, New York.

EXERCISE 2: MEASURING LIQUIDS

Procedure

1. Select the appropriate measuring utensils.
2. Place the container on a level surface. Carefully pour the liquid into the container. Your eye should be level with the measure mark and liquid added until the bottom of the meniscus rests on the mark.

EXERCISE 3: MEASURING SOLIDS

Procedure

1. Weigh the appropriate measuring utensil on an ounce scale.
2. For ***dry*** solids (e.g., granulated sugar, flour), lightly spoon the material into the container. For ***moist*** solids (e.g., brown sugar, solid fats), firmly pack the material into the container.
3. Reweigh the filled container on the scale, record the actual weight of the material.
4. Convert to metric equivalents; record on the table.
5. Compare and discuss variability of weights recorded by class members for the same measure.

Food	Measure	Weight oz./g
Dry solid		
	1 tsp (5 mL)	
	1 tbsp (15 mL)	
	1 cup (240 mL)	
Moist solid		
	1 tsp (5 mL)	
	1 tbsp (15 mL)	
	1 cup (240 mL)	

Note: The same measure of different foods does not yield the same weight.

EXERCISE 4: CLEANUP

PROCEDURE

Observe procedures to be followed in cleanup of utensils, stoves, and kitchen unit. Consider appropriate disposal of waste to facilitate recycling.

SUMMARY QUESTIONS—MEASUREMENTS, USE OF INGREDIENTS, AND LABORATORY TECHNIQUES

1. Given ⅔ cup (160 mL) hydrogenated shortening, what type of measuring equipment is used?

2. How does the technique for measuring solid fat differ from such solid ingredients as baking powder and sugar?

3. When measuring 5 tbsp (75 mL) of milk, what equipment would be most accurate?

4. In measuring ⅜ cup (90 mL) of flour, what equipment should be used?

5. In a recipe that calls for 3 cups (720 mL) sugar, how much (in pounds, grams) will need to be purchased?

6. Regarding stick margarine:
   a. What is the easiest way to measure ^{3}¾ cup (180 mL)? ¼ cup (60 mL)?

   b. ½ cup (120 mL) margarine is equal to how much of a pound? How many grams?

7. A recipe requires 7 cups (1680 mL) all-purpose flour; ¾ lb. (340.5 g) is available. How much more will need to be purchased? In pounds? In grams?

Reminder: In the lab you will not consume a full portion of the products you prepare; however, be able to identify the correct portion sizes of any assigned products.

Portions

Standard FDA serving sizes are found on food product labels and/or in the following document: http://vm.cfsan.fda.gov/~lrd/cf101-12.html. Go to Table 2—*Reference Amounts Customarily Consumed Per Eating Occasion*.

LAB POLICIES AND PROCEDURES

PERSONAL HYGIENE:

- Wash hands often!
- Wear flat, closed-toe shoes.
- Wear a hair restraint or tie hair off face.
- Wear a lab coat.
- During preparation, taste food with a utensil and small plate. Do not use fingers to taste foods; use utensils!
- No eating or drinking in the food preparation areas.
- **Other:**

LAB USE:

- Wash food preparation surfaces prior to use.
- In the interest of energy conservation, ovens should not be set until necessary. Instructions to set the oven are provided at the ***beginning*** of recipes to serve as a reminder to set the oven.
- Avoid food spills; clean as often as necessary.
- Beware of sharp knives left in the water in the sinks.
- Beware of burns from hot foods.
- Do not use cell phones in the lab.
- **Other:**

FOOD SAFETY:

- Follow proper cooking and holding temperatures (also see Appendix H).
- Avoid cross-contamination and observe personal hygiene and cleanliness procedures as stated above.
- **Other:**

Food Allergies:

- Be aware of possible food allergens used as ingredients in food preparation.
- Become knowledgeable about ingredient alternatives useful in a recipe.
- Consult with a healthcare provider to manage any personal food allergies.
- **Other:**

Have fun!

B. Cereal and Starch

Words do not make flour.

— Italian proverb

OBJECTIVES

To define and explain the role of separating agents in starch cookery

To describe the events that occur in starch cookery, their relationship to temperature, thickness, and flavor of the product

To delineate the effect of sugar and acid on starch-thickened products

To recognize individual properties of flour and cornstarch

To relate principles of starch cookery to the preparation of cereal products, including "convenience" foods

To relate principles of starch cookery to a variety of starch-thickened products

To identify cereal and starch allergens and acceptable recipe alternatives

To prepare a palatable starch product, delineating and giving reasons for each step

To appraise the nutritive, sanitary, and economic dimensions of starch and cereal products

Baked products—batters and dough—are discussed in another chapter.

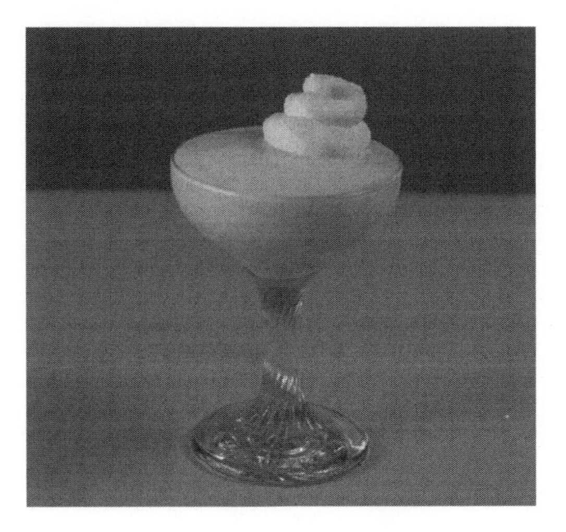

STARCH-THICKENED PUDDING.
Courtesy: SYSCO® Incorporated.

REFERENCES[1]

Appendix E
www.grainpower.org
www.MyPyramid.gov
www.wheatfoods.org
http://www.ncaur.usda.gov/cpf/trimtech.html
www.celiac.com
www.csaceliacs.org
www.gluten.net (GIG)

[1] Websites current at time of printing.

www.msrecoverydiet.com

http://www.eatright.org/cps/rde/xchg/ada/hs.xsl/nutrition_16994_ENU_HTML.htm

http://www.webmd.com/diet/guide/gluten-intolerance-against-grain

http://www.webmd.com/digestive-disorders/celiac-disease/features/gluten-intolerance-against-grain

Case, S. 2006. *Gluten-Free Diet. A Comprehensive Resource Guide*. Case Nutrition Consulting, Regina, Saskatchewan, Canada.

Terms

Absorption
Adsorption
Amylopectin
Amylose
Bran
Colloidal dispersion
Endosperm
Enriched
Germ
Gelation
Gelatinization
Gluten-free
Granule/grain
Imbibition
Intolerance/allergy
Maltodextrin
Modified starch
Polymer
Separating agent
Sol/gel
Starch
Suspension
Viscosity

BOX 1: STANDARD PROCEDURE

Flour/Cornstarch-Thickened Product

(Reference for Exercises 1 to 3)

1. In a saucepan, mix the starch and separating agent (melted fat, sugar, cold liquid).
2. Slowly add remaining liquid, stirring constantly.
3. Cook, stirring constantly until mixture boils.
4. Cook a few minutes longer to improve flavor, stirring gently.

EXERCISE 1: SEPARATION OF STARCH GRANULES

Procedure

1. Prepare a starch-thickened product following the standard procedure (Box 1) and using the proportions of ingredients listed in the table below.
2. Evaluate the consistency of hot products using the palatability terms provided in Box 2.

Starch	Separating Agent	Boiling Water	Hot—Palatability
1 tbsp (15 mL) flour	None	½ cup (120 mL)	
1 tbsp (15 mL) flour	1 tbsp (15 mL) melted fat	½ cup (120 mL)	
1 tbsp (15 mL) flour	¼ cup (60 mL) cold water	¼ cup (60 mL)	
1 tbsp (15 mL) flour	1 tbsp (15 mL) sugar	½ cup (120 mL)	

1. What is the scientific explanation for lump formation?

2. Explain how the following function as separating agents:
   a. Melted fat

   b. Cold liquid

   c. Sugar

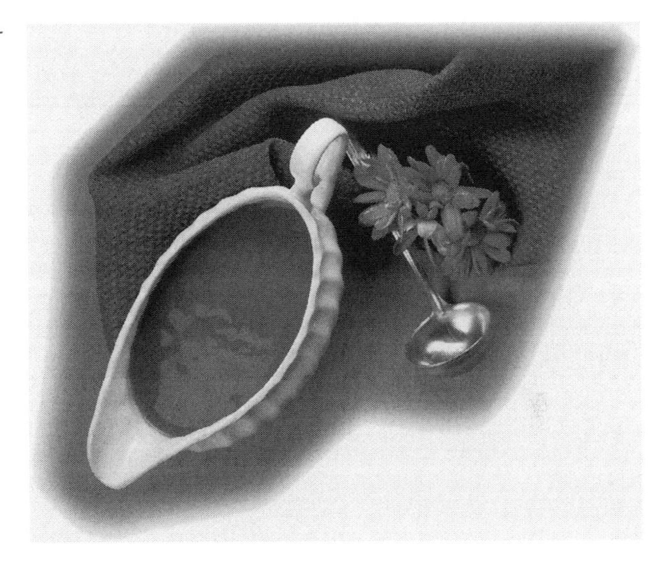

STARCH-THICKENED GRAVY.
Courtesy: SYSCO® Incorporated.

BOX 2: PALATABILITY TERMS

EXERCISES 1 TO 3

APPEARANCE	TEXTURE	FLAVOR	CONSISTENCY
Opaque	Lumpy	Raw	Thin
Cloudy	Fairly smooth	Cooked	Medium thick
Translucent	Smooth		Thick
Transparent			Gel-like

EXERCISE 2: PROPERTIES OF WHEAT AND CORNSTARCH

PROCEDURE

1. Prepare a starch-thickened sauce with each of the starches listed by following the standard procedure (Box 1). Use ¼ cup (60 mL) cold water as the separating agent, then add ¾ cup (180 mL) water.
2. Record observations regarding consistency and appearance of sauces while hot and after cooling, using terms provided.
3. Save the hot and cool samples of the cornstarch mixture to use as the standard in Exercise 3.

Starch	Observations of Consistency, Appearance	
	Hot Sauce	Cooled Sauce
2 tbsp (30 mL) cornstarch (standard)		
2 tbsp (30 mL) flour		
2 tbsp (30 mL) browned flour[a]		

[a] To brown, spread flour in a thin layer in a flat pan. Bake at 375°F (190°C), stirring frequently, until flour is light brown.

1. Draw a diagram or describe:
   a. Starch in cold water

   b. Starch–water mixture heated to boiling

   c. Cooked mixture cooled to refrigeration temperature

2. Explain, using scientific terms, how a starch ***gel*** is formed from a starch *sol*.

3. What factor(s) determine the type of separating agent to be used in a starch-thickened product?

4. How could the same thickness in a final product be obtained if a recipe listed 1 tbsp (15 mL) flour and only cornstarch was available for use due to food allergies?

5. Why is a flour product cooked for additional time after maximum thickness is reached?

EXERCISE 3: EFFECT OF SUGAR AND ACID ON GELATINIZATION

PROCEDURE

1. Prepare a starch-thickened sauce following the standard procedure, with 2 tbsp (30 mL) cornstarch, and using the proportions of ingredients listed below. (Cook the vinegar mixture slowly.)
2. Evaluate the consistency of hot and cooled sauces compared to the standard in Exercise 2.
3. Record observations as to consistency of hot and cold products.

		Observations	
Separating Agent	Water	Hot Sauce	Cooled Sauce
½ cup (120 mL) sugar	1 cup (240 mL)		
¼ cup (60 mL) vinegar	¾ cup (180 mL)		
¼ cup (60 mL) water	½ cup (120 mL) + ¼ cup (60 mL) vinegar (added after thick)		

1. Explain how large amounts of sugar affect the gelatinization of starch and characteristics of the sol/gel.

2. Explain how acid affects the gelatinization of starch. How does the time of acid addition affect product results?

3. Based on these experiments, when should lemon juice be added to a lemon pie filling mixture?

EXERCISE 4: APPLICATION OF PRINCIPLES TO STARCH-THICKENED PRODUCTS

PROCEDURE

1. Prepare a starch-thickened product from the assigned list of ingredients (no recipe). Based on previous experiments and readings, outline procedures, giving scientific reasons for each step.
2. Show the gravy to your instructor.

NAME OF PRODUCT:	
Steps	Explanation

3. Evaluation: Analyze success or failure of the product, based on scientific principles.

	Explanation
Texture:	
Consistency:	

4. Evaluate all recipes of test products, noting types of separating agents used and general palatability.

Recipe Ingredients[a]						Evaluation
CHEESE SAUCE						
1 cup	240 mL	milk	⅓ cup	80 mL	processed cheese	
dash	30 mL	paprika	2 tbsp	30 mL	flour	
2 tbsp		margarine				
CORN CHOWDER						
2 tbsp	30 mL	finely chopped onion	1 cup	240 mL	milk	
		margarine	1	120 mL	chicken bouillon cube	
2 tbsp	30 mL	flour			creamed corn	
1 tbsp	15 mL		½ cup			

Recipe Ingredients[a]						Evaluation
CREAM OF POTATO SOUP						
1½ cups	360 mL	milk	½ tbsp	7.5 mL	pimento, chopped	
1 tbsp	15 mL	margarine			diced cooked	
1 tbsp	15 mL	flour	1 cup	240 mL	potatoes	
RAISIN SAUCE FOR MEAT						
½ cup	120 mL	brown sugar	2 tbsp	30 mL	lemon juice	
1 tsp	5 mL	dry mustard[b]	¼ tsp	1.25 mL	grated lemon rind	
2 tbsp	30 mL	flour	1½ cups	360 mL	water	
2 tbsp	30 mL	vinegar	⅓ cup	80 mL	raisins	
TOMATO SAUCE						
1 tbsp	15 mL	green pepper, chopped	1 tbsp	15 mL	cornstarch	
1 tsp	5 mL	grated onion	1 cup	240 ml	tomato juice	
1 tbsp	15 mL	margarine				
FRUIT SAUCE						
2 tbsp	30 mL	margarine	2 tbsp	30 mL	lemon juice	
¾ cup	180 mL	confectioner's sugar	2 tsp	10 mL	orange juice	
2 tbsp	30 mL	cornstarch	⅓ cup	80 mL	orange rind	
½ cup	120 mL	water				
LEMON SAUCE						
1 tbsp	15 mL	cornstarch	¼ cup	60 mL	lemon juice	
¾ cup	180 mL	water	¼ tsp	1.25 mL	grated lemon rind	
⅓ cup	80 mL	sugar	dash		nutmeg	
1 tbsp	15 mL	margarine				
PUDDING, BUTTERSCOTCH[c]						
1 cup	240 mL	milk	1 tbsp	15 mL	margarine	Microwave[c]:
⅓ cup	80 mL	brown sugar, packed	2 tbsp	30 mL	cornstarch	
½ tsp	2.5 mL	vanilla				
PUDDING, CHOCOLATE[c]						
¼ cup	60 mL	sugar	½ tsp	2.5 mL	vanilla	Microwave[c]:
1½ tbsp	22.5 mL	cornstarch	½ square		unsweetened chocolate, grated	
1 cup	240 mL	milk				
1 tbsp	15 mL	margarine				
Pudding, instant						
Pudding, microwave						

(continued on next page)

Recipe Ingredients[a]						Evaluation
SWEET-SOUR SAUCE						
½ cup	120 mL	pineapple juice	½ tsp	2.5 mL	prepared mustard[b]	
1 tbsp	15 mL	vinegar	1 tbsp	15 ml	cornstarch	
2 tbsp	30 mL	brown sugar	¼ cup	60 mL	water	
½ tsp	2.5 mL	paprika	½ cup	120 mL	pineapple tidbits	
1		chicken bouillon cube	¼ cup	60 mL	green pepper, chopped	

[a] Circle separating agent used (only one).

[b] Treat mustard as starch.

[c] See chapter on Microwave Cooking for microwave recipes.

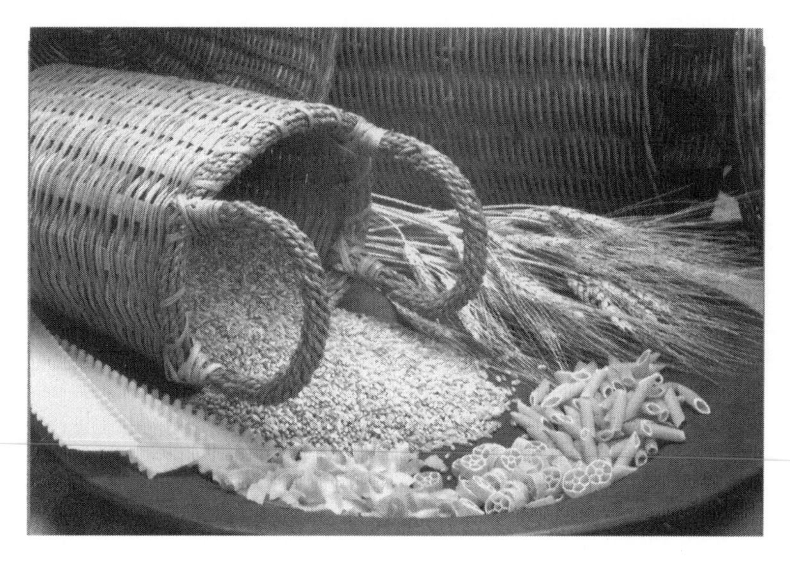

GRAINS.

Courtesy: Wheat Foods Council.

EXERCISE 5: PREPARING CEREAL PRODUCTS

PROCEDURE

1. Cook ¼ cup (60 mL) cereal product as directed, unless otherwise assigned.
2. Measure, record yield, and display.
3. Record palatability assessments of all products using the following palatability terms.

PALATABILITY TERMS		
TEXTURE	CONSISTENCY	FLAVOR
Smooth	Thick	Sweet
Lumpy	Thin	Nutty
Grainy	Gel-like	Raw starch
	Gummy	
	Sticky	

Cooking Directions for Cereals/Grain Products

Granular or finely milled grains—cornmeal, farina, grits. Add grains to cold water. Boil gently. Stir occasionally.

Whole or coarsely milled grains—barley, buckwheat (kasha), bulgur, rice, oats. Add grains to boiling water. Boil gently. Add water as needed.

Pasta—Add to boiling water. Boil uncovered, until desired tenderness is achieved. To prevent boiling over, add ½ tsp (2.5 mL) oil to cooking water.

Evaluation of Cereal Products

Grain ¼ cup (60 mL)	Water[a] (cup, mL)	Cooking Time (min)	Cooked Yield	Palatability Characteristics
GRANULAR/FINE				
Farina	1½ cups (360 mL)	3–5		
Cornmeal	1½ cups (360 mL)	3–5		
Cornmeal grits	¾ cup (180 mL)	5		
FLAKED/COARSE				
Oatmeal, regular	¾ cup (180 mL)	15		
Oatmeal, quick	¾ cup (180 mL)	2		
Oatmeal, quick	¾ cup (180 mL)	2 min, stir while cooking; + 5 min		
Oatmeal, instant	Package directions			
WHOLE/COARSE				
Rice, regular	½ cup (120 mL)	15–20		
Rice, brown	½ cup (120 mL)	40		
Rice, instant	¼ cup (60 mL)	Boiling water over rice, let stand 5 min		

(continued on next page)

Evaluation of Cereal Products

Grain ¼ cup (60 mL)	Water[a] (cup, mL)	Cooking Time (min)	Cooked Yield	Palatability Characteristics
OTHER GRAINS[b]				
Wheat bulgur	1 cup (240 mL)	15		
Wheat bulgur	½ cup (120 mL)	Cold water, soak 10 min		
Barley, quick-cook	½ cup (120 mL)	15		
Buckwheat (kasha)	½ cup (120 mL)	15		
Buckwheat (kasha) ½ cup	Package directions; use ½ egg			
Couscous (semolina)	¼ cup (60 mL) boiling water	Soak 5 min		
Quinoa	Package directions			
PASTA				
Pasta	1 pt. (480 mL)	7–12		
Whole wheat pasta	1 pt. (480 mL)	7–12		
Gluten-Free pasta	See package			

[a] With long-cooking grains, for example, brown rice, additional water may have to be added during cooking.
[b] Experiment with other grains, for example, millet and quinoa (*keen-wa*).

CEREAL RECIPES[2]

Barley Cheese Casserole

water	3 cups	720 mL	margarine	2 tbsp	30 mL
quick pearled barley	1 cup	240 mL	cooked tomatoes, drained	2 cups	480 mL
finely chopped onion	¼ cup	60 ml	cheese, grated	2 oz.	57 g

1. Set oven at 350°F (175°C).
2. Add barley to boiling water. Cover and simmer 10 to 12 minutes until barley is tender. Stir occasionally. Drain.
3. Sauté onion in fat until tender.
4. Add onion and remaining ingredients to greased casserole.
5. Bake 10 to 15 minutes until casserole is heated through or reheat in a frying pan on top of stove. Season. (3 to 4 servings.)

[2] Recipes may contain known allergens. See Appendix E.

Cheesy Corn Grits

quick-cooking grits	½ cup	120 mL	milk	⅓ cup	80 mL
milk	1½ cups	360 mL	cheese, grated	½ cup	120 mL
egg, slightly beaten	1		chives	2 tbsp	30 mL

1. Boil grits in milk.
2. Add remaining ingredients and place in small greased casserole. Bake at 350°F (175°C) 35 to 40 minutes. (2 to 3 servings.)

Fiesta Rice

water	2 cups	480 mL	chopped pimento	1 tbsp	15 mL
rice	1 cup	240 mL	chili powder	¼ tsp	1.25 mL
margarine	1 tbsp	15 mL	drained cooked tomatoes	½ cup	120 mL
chopped green pepper	2 tbsp	30 mL			

1. Cook rice in unsalted water about 18 minutes. Drain and keep hot.
2. Sauté pepper and pimento in fat until softened. Stir in chili powder and tomatoes.
3. Combine hot vegetable mixture and rice. Reheat. (2 servings.)

Macaroni and Cheese

macaroni	½ cup	120 mL	dry mustard	⅛ tsp	0.63 mL
chopped onion	¼ cup	60 mL	pepper	⅛ tsp	0.63 mL
margarine	1 tbsp	15 mL	milk	1 cup	240 mL
flour	1 tsp	5 mL	processed American cheese	1 cup	240 mL

1. Cook macaroni in large amount of water until just tender. Drain.
2. In a medium saucepan, sauté onion until tender. Add flour and seasonings. Stir in milk.
3. Cook over medium heat, stirring until thickened. Reduce heat; add cheese and macaroni. Stir. Let stand 5 minutes. (2 servings.)

Variation: Add 1 cup (240 mL) cooked vegetable with cheese.

Pasta Primavera

thin noodles	1 cup	240 mL	garlic powder	dash	dash
broccoli florets	¼ cup	60 mL	vegetable oil	½ tsp	2.5 mL
carrots, diced	¼ cup	60 mL	cornstarch	1 tsp	5 mL
red onion, sliced	¼ cup	60 mL	margarine	½ tsp	2.5 mL
green pepper strips	1 tbsp	15 mL	milk or water	⅓ cup	80 mL
basil leaves	¼ tsp	1.25 mL			

1. Cook noodles according to package directions. Drain.
2. Stir fry fresh vegetables and seasonings in oil, lifting and turning, until vegetables are tender crisp. Remove vegetables from pan.
3. Mix cornstarch with milk. Add with margarine in fry pan. Slowly heat, stirring constantly, until thickened. (Sauce will be thin.)
4. Add sauce and vegetables to noodles, mix gently. Heat to serving temperature. (2 servings.)

Pasta Salad

pasta, penne	4 oz.	114 g	onion, minced	2 tbsp	30 mL
broccoli florets	½ cup	120 mL	garlic, minced	1 tsp	5 mL
carrots, diced	¼ cup	60 mL	Italian dressing	¼ cup	60 mL
black olives, sliced	½ cup	120 mL	Dijon mustard	½ tsp	2.5 mL

1. Boil pasta as directed on package. Drain and allow to cool.
2. Steam broccoli and carrots until tender crisp. Cool.
3. Combine all ingredients, tossing well. Refrigerate. (2 to 4 servings.)

Polenta

coarse cornmeal	½ cup	120 mL	paprika	⅛ tsp	0.63 mL
water, boiling	2 cups	480 mL	grated cheese	¼ cup	60 mL

1. Slowly add cornmeal to boiling water.
2. Cook, stirring frequently, over low heat about 15 minutes, or until thickened (or this may be cooked in the top of a double boiler over boiling water).
3. Pour hot mixture into 7-inch (18-cm) pie pan or small cake pan.
4. Sprinkle with paprika and cheese. Cover and refrigerate. If desired, reheat before serving. Note: Serve plain on a plate, top with spaghetti or pizza sauce or sautéed green peppers and onions. (3 servings.)

QUINOA-VEGETABLE MEDLEY

quinoa	1 cup	240 mL	finely chopped	½ cup	120 mL
cold water	2 cups	480 mL	onion	½ cup	120 mL
olive oil	1 tbsp	15 mL	finely chopped	½ cup	120 mL
zucchini, chopped	1 cup	240 mL	bell pepper	1 tbsp	15 mL
mushrooms, chopped	½ cup	120 mL	tomato, chopped		
			balsamic vinegar		

1. Boil water and add quinoa. Reduce heat to low and continue to cook quinoa for 20 minutes.
2. Sauté the vegetables except the tomato for 5 minutes.
3. Add tomatoes and vinegar. Heat through.
4. Combine the cooked quinoa and vegetables. Season. (4 to 6 servings.)

RICE PUDDING

cooked rice/leftover rice	1 cup	240 mL	vanilla	½ tsp	2.5 mL
milk	1¼ cups	300 mL	lemon peel	dash	2.5 mL
sugar	2 tbsp	30 mL	lemon juice	½ tsp	30 mL
egg, slightly beaten	1		raisins	2 tbsp	

1. Set oven to 325°F (165°C).
2. Combine all ingredients and pour into greased casserole.
3. Bake 45 minutes. (3 to 4 servings.)

TABOULEH

bulgur	½ cup	120 mL	finely chopped, seeded cucumber	½ cup	120 mL
cold water	1 cup	240 mL	finely chopped bell pepper	½ cup	120 mL
finely chopped tomato	1		fresh lemon juice	⅓ cup	80 mL
finely chopped parsley	1 cup	240 mlL	olive oil	2 tbsp	30 mL
finely chopped scallions	½ cup	120 mL			

1. Place bulgur and water in a bowl, and refrigerate 1 hour. Drain if necessary.
2. Combine remaining ingredients. Add to bulgur, stirring to blend. Refrigerate.
3. Before serving, stir salad and adjust seasoning. (6 servings.)

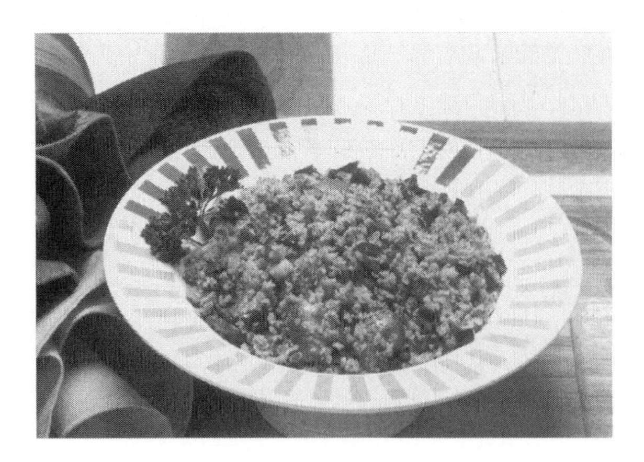

BULGAR.
Courtesy: Wheat Foods Council.

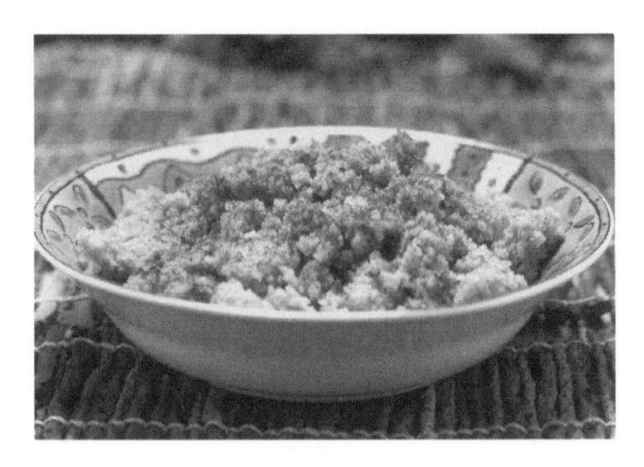

COUSCOUS.
Courtesy: Wheat Foods Council.

Evaluation—Cereal Recipes	
Cereal Recipe	Palatability (see terms)
Other:	
Other:	
Other:	

SUMMARY QUESTIONS—CEREAL AND STARCH

Starches

1. A fruit sauce recipe calls for 3 tbsp (45 mL) cornstarch. For a successful recipe, how much sugar would be needed as a separating agent? How much fat? How much cold liquid?

2. When preparing a sauce or gravy, when will maximum thickness be observed? How can the thickness of hot gravy be increased if it is necessary?

3. How does the starch in "instant" pudding differ from the starch used in "homemade" forms?

4. How are modified starches and maltodextrins used in the food industry? Explain.

5. Why are prepared creamed (milk-thickened sauce) foods and meat gravies frequently considered a food-safety risk after they are prepared?

Cereals

1. What are the desired palatability characteristics of a cooked grain product?

2. What is the major problem encountered in cooking finely milled grains to achieve a smooth texture? How is this problem resolved?

3. How and why does excessive stirring affect palatability of cereal grains?

4. What are the advantages and disadvantages of cooking cereal products in the top of a double boiler, over boiling water?

5. How does *instant* rice differ from *regular, long-cooking* rice?

6. How is rice enriched? Should enriched rice be rinsed before cooking? Explain.

7. Complete the table for one serving by reading labels or using appropriate references.

Product	Energy (kcal)	Protein (g)	Cholesterol (g)	Ca (%)	Iron (%)	Thiamin (mg)	Riboflavin (mg)
Rice, enriched							
Macaroni, enriched							
Grits, regular, unenriched							
Grits, instant, enriched							
Couscous							

8. Identify the contribution that cereals make to the fiber content of diets.

9. Describe proper storage of whole grains.

10. Identify the costs of various rice products:

Product	Cost/Package	Package Size	Portion Cost
Long-cooking rice			
Long-cooking rice, flavored			
Instant rice			
Microwave rice			

11. List several "convenience" cereal and starch products such as sauces and gravies, and how they are used.

12. Identify how to accommodate food allergies in recipes involving cereals and starches.

13. Identify the nutritional effect of eating a ready-to-eat variety of breakfast cereal vs. cooked cereal.

14. Describe nutritional advantages of cooking with whole grains.

15. Differentiate between a food intolerance and a food allergy.

Dietitian's Note

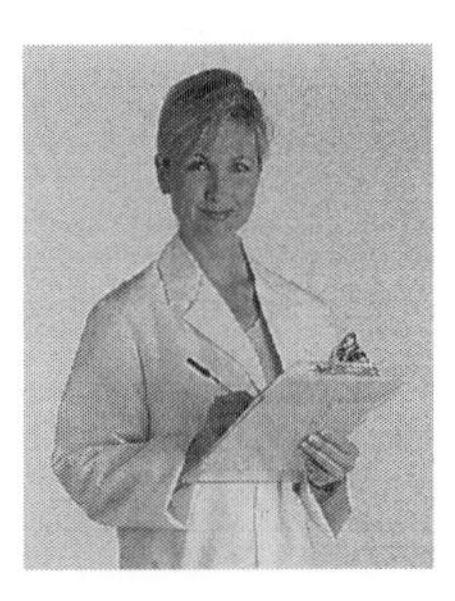

Gluten-Free Modified Diet

See references.

www.vegsoc.org — search Gluten-free. Then, search for the Information Sheet that contains:

Food	Gluten-Free	Gluten-Containing
Cereals, flours, cakes, biscuits	Arrowroot, buckwheat, corn/maize, potato flour, rice, sago, tapioca, soy	Wheat, oats[a], rye, barley[b]

[a] Oats do not contain gluten; however, they may become cross-contaminated in processing or shipping.

[b] Barley or barley extract may be in food products, thus read labels.

Allergens may also include milk, egg, and other foods appearing in recipes. See Appendix E.

C. Fruits and Vegetables

Vegetables are a must on a diet.
I suggest carrot cake, zucchini bread, and pumpkin pie.

— ***Garfield*, Jim Davis**

Objectives

To know and describe parts of the parenchyma cell and how these are affected by heat
To relate cellular structure and principles of osmosis to recrisping vegetables
To evaluate the effect of processing on the sugar content of vegetables
To relate nutrient losses to changes in the structure of a plant cell during processing
To describe the effects of pH on the color characteristics of raw fruits
To compare the effectiveness of various factors in preventing enzymatic browning in fruits
To evaluate the effects of cooking procedures on the texture of cooked fruits
To know and describe the effect of pH changes on the color and texture of vegetables
To evaluate the effect of cooking procedures on the color, flavor, and texture of vegetables
To identify the role of convenience products in vegetable and fruit consumption
To illustrate palatable combinations of vegetables, noting contrasts in flavor, color, and texture
To demonstrate the ability to apply principles of vegetable cookery by preparing various vegetable items
To appraise the nutritive, economic, and sanitary dimensions of fruits and vegetables
To identify fruit and vegetable allergens and acceptable recipe modifications

References

Appendices E, K, M, N
www.5aday.gov; www.5aday.org
http://www.dole5aday.com
www.cancer.org
http://www.beef.org/ncbanutrition.aspx#
Gollman, B. and K. Pierce. 1998. *The Phytopia Cookbook: A World of Plant-Centered Cuisine*. Dallas, TX: Phytopia, Inc.
Seinfeld, J. 2007. *Deceptively Delicious: Simple Secrets to Get Your Kids Eating Good Food*. New York: Melcher Media.

Terms

Allium
Anthocyanin
Anthoxanthin
Bake
Brassica
Carotene
Cell membrane
Cell sap
Cellulose
Chlorophyll
Chop
Cytoplasm
Dice
Diffusion
Enzymatic browning
Enzyme
Glaze
Mince
Nucleus
Osmosis
Panned
Parenchyma
Pectic substances
Permeable
Plastid
Polyphenol
Semipermeable
Solute
Solution
Solvent
Substrate
Succulent
Tannin
Turgor
Vacuole

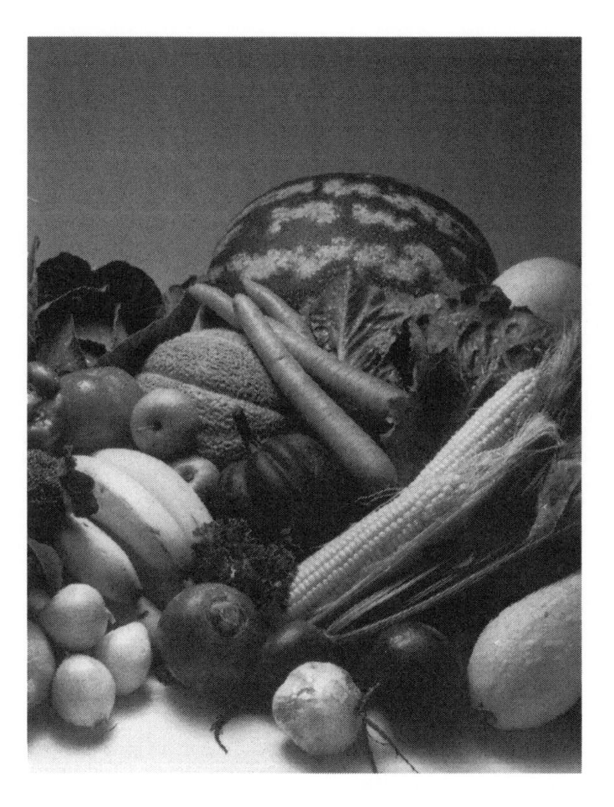

Fruits and Vegetables.
Courtesy: United Fresh Fruit and Vegetable Association.

EXERCISE 1: PROPERTIES OF PARENCHYMA CELLS

A. Components of Parenchyma Cell

1. Label parts of the parenchyma cell.

2. Identify fat- and water-soluble cell components.

3. List the major components of cell sap.

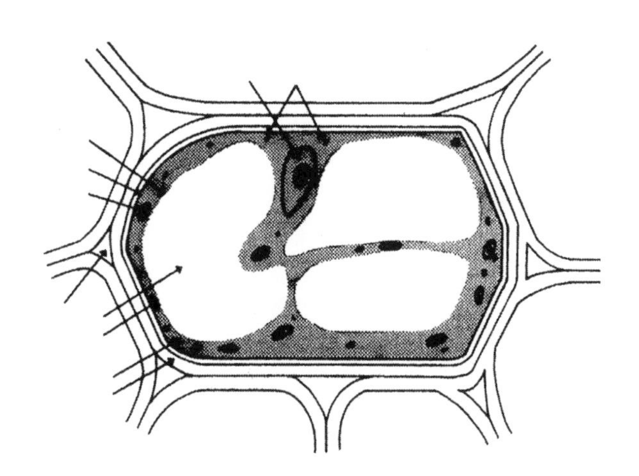

Parenchyma Cell.
Source: Division of Nutritional Sciences, New York State College of Human Ecology at Cornell, Ithaca, New York.

4. What is the effect on vacuole components of cutting through a cell (chopping, mashing)?

5. When living parenchyma cells are placed in water, how is the material in the vacuole affected? Why?

6. What changes in cell structure occur when a plant food is cooked?

7. When parenchyma cells are cooked in water, how is the material in the vacuole affected? What losses would you expect? Why?

8. Define and distinguish between *osmosis* and *diffusion*.

B. Recrisping Succulents

Procedure

1. For each treatment, process ½ cup (120 mL) limp celery as directed.
2. Record observations as to crispness and turgor after holding 2 hours.

Treatment	Observations
1 cup (240 mL) tap water	
1 cup (240 mL) salt solution (3 tbsp [45 mL] salt/1 cup [240 mL] water)	

1. Why is a solution of salt and water used, and not a mixture?

2. Based on these observations, what is the most effective method of recrisping vegetables?

3. Explain, using scientific principles and a diagram, the process of recrisping.

4. In vegetables that are recrisped for a long time would nutrient losses be expected? Explain.

5. List several vegetables that can be recrisped.

6. What storage methods keep vegetables crisp and eliminate the need for recrisping?

7. Based on these experiments, predict what would happen to raw peach slices sprinkled with sugar. Explain.

EXERCISE 2: FRUITS

A. Enzymatic Browning

Procedure

1. Prepare test solutions as indicated on the chart, prior to cutting fruit.
2. Test pH using Alkacid test paper.[1]
3. Peel assigned fruit (e.g., apples, bananas) and cut into 14 uniform slices.
4. For each treatment, use two fruit slices and thoroughly coat with test solutions. Leave two slices untreated.
5. Expose all fruit slices to air for 30 minutes. Record observations as to any color changes.
6. Summarize your conclusions regarding the most effective way to prevent enzymatic browning.

Test Solution	pH	Color after Exposure to Air	Explanation
Untreated			
¼ cup (60 mL) lemon juice			
¼ cup (60 mL) pineapple juice			
¼ cup (60 mL) water + 2 tbsp (30 mL) sugar			
¼ cup (60 mL) water + ¼ tsp (1.25 mL) cream of tartar			
¼ cup (60 mL) water + ⅛ tsp (0.63 mL) Fruit Fresh®			
¼ cup (60 mL) water + ⅛ tsp (0.63 mL) ascorbic acid			

[1] Test paper obtained from Fisher Scientific Co., Rochester, New York.

1. What components must be present for a fresh fruit or vegetable to brown?

2. What additives are used commercially to prevent browning of fresh/dried fruits? Potatoes?

B. Effect of Sugar on Texture and Flavor of Cooked Fresh Fruit

Procedure

1. Prepare sugar solution as directed.
2. Place each solution in a small, shallow pan.
3. Peel, core, and cut 2 cooking apples to make 16 uniform pieces.
4. Place 4 slices in each pan and cook covered (submerged) for 6 to 8 minutes over medium heat (more than the ½ cup of water may be necessary.)
5. Record a check mark for the *primary* movement of water and/or solutes that takes place in cooking.
6. Use palatability terms below and account for palatability characteristics that were observed.

Test Solution	Osmosis	Diffusion	Palatability	Explanation
½ cup (120 mL) water				
½ cup (120 mL) water + 2 tbsp (30 mL) sugar				
½ cup (120 mL) water + 1 cup (240 mL) sugar				
½ cup (120 mL) water; cook 6 min, then + 1 cup (240 mL) sugar; cook 2 min				

PALATABILITY TERMS

TEXTURE	FLAVOR	SHAPE
Firm	Uniform sweetness	Retains shape
Soft	Surface sweetness	Sauce
Mushy	Retains natural flavor	Shrunken
Glazed	Bland	

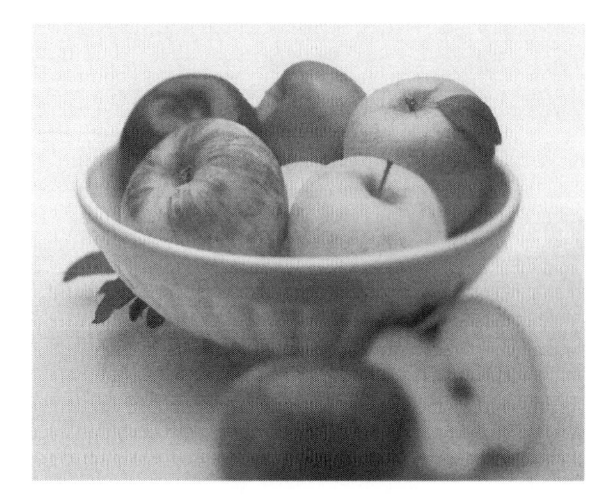

APPLES.
Courtesy: SYSCO® Incorporated.

1. Under what conditions does osmosis cease?

2. Are nutrients lost from fruit during osmosis? Explain.

3. Are nutrients lost from fruit during diffusion? Explain.

4. What are the effects of large amounts of sugar on plant pectins?

C. Effect of Sugar on Texture and Flavor of Cooked Dried Fruit

Procedure

1. Cook dried fruits in boiling test solution for 10 minutes.
2. Record observations and account for palatability.

Test Solution[a]	Palatability	Explanation
¼ cup (60 mL) raisins + ⅓ cup (80 mL) water		
¼ cup (60 mL) raisins + ⅓ cup (80 mL) water + ¼ cup (60 mL) sugar		

[a] Check to maintain sufficient test solution in saucepan.

Conclusions:

1. How does drying affect plant membranes?

2. What process occurs during the cooking of dried fruits?

D. Factors Affecting Anthocyanin Pigments

Procedures

1. Mix 2 tbsp (30 mL) assigned fruit juice (e.g., grape, blackberry, or cranberry) with each variable.
2. Record and explain results on chart.
3. Summarize conclusions.

Variable	Color	Explanation
1 tbsp (15 mL) lemon juice		
2 tbsp (30 mL) orange juice		
2 tbsp (30 mL) pineapple juice		
2 tbsp (30 mL) strong tea		
¼ tsp (1.25 mL) baking soda		
Iron chloride (few drops)		

Conclusions:

1. Is enzymatic browning a problem in the following? Explain.
   a. Canned apple slices

   b. Pear slices wrapped in plastic wrap

   c. Fresh fruit cup (grapes, cheese cubes, bananas)

2. Why do some fruits (apples, pears, bananas) turn brown when sliced or bruised, but the intact fruit does not brown?

3. To achieve a palatable cooked product (soft, sweet, tender) from a mixture of dried fruits, how should they be prepared? Why?

4. Provide examples of how one would apply information about reaction of anthocyanin pigments when working with whole fruits or juice mixtures.

5. What are the major nutrient contributions of fruits? Specify which fruits are not excellent sources of vitamin C.

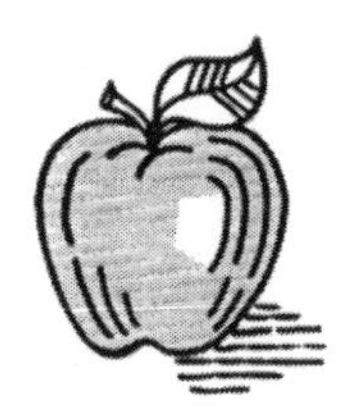

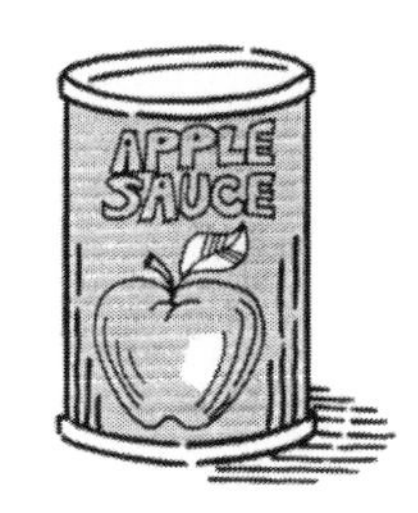

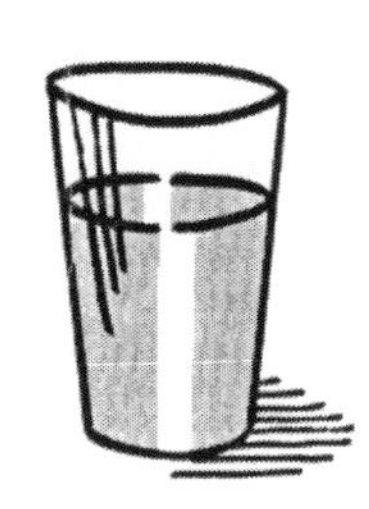

Whole apple with peel: 3.6 g fiber   Applesauce, ½ cup: 2.1 g fiber   Apple juice, ¾ cup: 0.2 g fiber

6. Explain how color can give an indication of the relative amounts of vitamin A in a fruit.

7. Account for the different values for fiber in the three apple products shown. What components of the whole apple contribute fiber?

8. Complete the following nutritive value chart:

Fruit	Energy (kcal)	Iron (mg)	Vitamin A IU/RE	Vitamin C (mg)	Fiber (g)
Apple (1 medium)					
Apricots, dried (½ cup, 120 mL)					
Cantaloupe (¼)					
Grapefruit, pink (½)					
Grapefruit, white (½)					
Orange (1 medium)					
Pear (1 medium)					
Peach (1 medium)					
Peaches, canned (½ cup; 120 mL)					
Pineapple, canned (2 slices)					
Prunes, dried (½ cup; 120 mL)					
Prunes, stewed (½ cup; 120 mL)					
Strawberries (½ cup; 120 mL)					

9. Identify fruits or vegetables causing allergies (see Appendix E).

PALATABILITY TERMS

TEXTURE	COLOR	FLAVOR
Hard	Natural	Natural
Firm	Red-blue, green-blue, gray-blue	Bland
Crisp	Pink	Mild
Tender	Bright green, olive green	Strong
Soft	White, cream, yellow	Off-flavor
Mushy	Other (please describe)	Other (describe)

COOKING VEGETABLES— PIGMENTS, PALATABILITY, PRECAUTIONS

PIGMENTS

Green (chlorophyll)
- beet greens
- broccoli
- butter beans (lima beans)
- collards
- green beans
- green cabbage
- kale
- peas
- spinach
- Swiss chard

Yellow (carotene)
- carrots
- rutabagas
- summer squash
- sweet potatoes
- wax beans
- winter squash (Hubbard, butternut)
- yams
- yellow turnips

Red (anthocyanin)
- beets
- red cabbage

White (anthoxanthin)
- cauliflower
- onions
- white potato
- white turnip

FLAVOR

Allium spp.
- chive
- garlic
- leeks
- onion
- shallots

Brassica spp.
- broccoli
- Brussels sprouts
- cabbage
- cauliflower
- kale
- turnip
- rutabagas

Precautions

As a precaution against contamination and growth of harmful bacteria:[1]

- Carefully wash hands before handling fresh produce, and between cutting and eating fresh produce.
- Rinse produce to remove harmful bacteria prior to consumption (even uneaten, disposed-of rinds), and after removing outer leaves and peels.
- Prepare fruits and vegetables on sanitary work surfaces with sanitary utensils.
- When fruits and vegetables are cut, inadvertent contamination has occurred; therefore, cover and refrigerate during storage to slow any bacterial growth.

[1]Adapted from *Tufts University Diet & Nutrition Letter* 14(11):1–2, 1997.

EXERCISE 3: COOKING VEGETABLES[2]

A. Effect of pH on Pigments and Texture

Caution: Watch water levels in pot!

Procedure

1. Select vegetables characteristically colored by the pigments, as assigned (spinach, carrots, red cabbage, white potato). Each vegetable will be cooked three ways.
2. For each vegetable, peel (if necessary) and cut into uniformly sized pieces.
3. For each treatment place 1 cup (240 mL) assigned vegetable and ¾ cup (180 mL) boiling water in a small saucepan. Add soda or vinegar as assigned. Maintain sufficient water level at all times!
4. Measure pH of water using Alkacid test paper and record.
5. Cover pan and bring water back to a boil. Start timing the cooking.[3]
6. After 10 minutes, remove half of the vegetable. Label and display. Cook the remaining portion 15 more minutes. Drain, label, and display.

[2] All fruits and vegetables intended for consumption should be washed well prior to preparation and cooking.

[3] Check to maintain sufficient water in saucepan.

7. Compare the color and texture of all samples. Record observations.

Vegetable Treatment	pH	Cooked 10 minutes		Cooked 25 minutes	
		Color	Texture	Color	Texture
Chlorophyll water only (control)					
+ ½ tsp (2.5 mL) soda					
+ 2 tbsp (30 mL) vinegar					
Carotene water only					
+ ½ tsp (2.5 mL) soda					
+ 2 tbsp (30 mL) vinegar					
Anthocyanin water only					
+ ½ tsp (2.5 mL) soda					
+ 2 tbsp (30 mL) vinegar					
Anthoxanthin water only					
+ ½ tsp (2.5 mL) soda					
+ 2 tbsp (30 mL) vinegar					

B. Effect of Cooking Procedure on Pigments and Flavors

Caution: Watch water levels in pot!

Procedure

1. Select a vegetable characteristically colored by chlorophyll and anthocyanin pigments.
2. Select a vegetable from the *Allium* and *Brassica* families.
3. Prepare 1 cup (240 mL) vegetable for each variable. Follow directions in the table for *cover and amount of water*, cooking the same vegetable two different ways.
4. Add water; start timing after water returns to a boil. Maintain sufficient water level at all times!
5. Remove half of the vegetable after cooking 10 minutes. Label and display. Cook remaining portion 15 more minutes to make the 25-minute variable. Label and display.

6. Evaluate all vegetables, and record observations.

Pigment	Cover	Water[a]	Cooked 10 minutes		Cooked 25 minutes	
			Color	Texture	Color	Texture
Chlorophyll	On	½ cup (120 mL)				
Chlorophyll	Off	to cover				
Anthocyanin	On	½ cup (120 mL)				
Anthocyanin	Off	to cover				

Flavor	Cover	Water[a]	Color	Flavor	Color	Flavor
Allium	On	½ cup (120 mL)				
Allium	Off	to cover				
Brassica	On	½ cup (120 mL)				
Brassica	Off	to cover				

[a] Check to maintain sufficient water in saucepan.

1. Why was there no variable in which 1 cup (240 mL) of vegetable was cooked in ½ cup (120 mL) of water, with the cover "off"?

2. Predict the effect on flavor of a vegetable from the *Allium* family and one from the *Brassica* family if each had been cooked, covered with water, in a pan with a cover.

3. Summarize the effect of *long cooking time* on the factors listed below:

Factor/Variable	Effect of Time	Explanation
A. Texture		
B. Color		
Chlorophyll		
Carotene		
Anthocyanin		
Anthoxanthin		
C. Flavor		
Allium		
Brassica		
D. Nutritive Value		
Vitamin A		
Vitamin C		
Thiamin		

4. Summarize the effect of covering the pan when cooking the following:

Vegetable	Effect of Cover	Explanation
Green pigment		
Red pigment		
Allium flavor		
Brassica flavor		

C. Application of Principles to Cooking a Variety of Vegetables

Procedure

1. Examine the display of raw vegetables, observing characteristics that denote freshness and excellent quality. Consider percentage waste as vegetables are prepared.
2. Prepare assigned vegetable recipe and plan cooking times (item with longest estimated preparation and cooking time should be first) to serve the product in ____ hour(s). If assigned recipe is to be cooked in the microwave; refer to the vegetable section of the microwave chapter.

3. Evaluate the palatability of all products, and complete the chart on pigment, flavor, and palatability.
4. Calculate the nutritive value of *one* or more recipes as assigned.

Evaluation of Vegetable Recipes

Vegetable Recipe	Major Pigment	Major Flavor	Palatability (see terms)

Nutritive Value of Assigned Recipe(s)

Food	Measure	Energy (kcal)	Protein (g)	Calcium (mg)	Iron (mg)	Vitamin A (IU/RE)	Vitamin C (mg)	Thiamin (mg)	Riboflavin (mg)

VEGETABLE RECIPES[4–6]

BEETS

Panned Beets

1. Peel beets (1½ cups; 360 mL) and remove stems. Slice, dice, or shred the beets.
2. Heat 1 tbsp (15 mL) oil in a heavy skillet or saucepan.
3. Add beets and toss until the vegetable is coated with oil. Add a small amount of water if necessary. Turn the heat down and stir to prevent burning. Vegetable should be crisp in texture. (Two servings.)

BROCCOLI

1. Remove coarse leaves and tough parts of stalk.
2. Split stalks, peel if tough; leave 3-inch (7.5-cm) stem on florets.
3. Boil uncovered in a small amount of water for 3 minutes. Cover, cook 5 to 8 minutes longer until just tender. Drain.
4. If desired, add 1 tsp (5 mL) margarine to each cup (240 mL) cooked vegetable; mix lightly. Season.

Steamed Broccoli Medley

bay leaf	1	240 mL	cauliflower pieces	1 cup	240 mL
broccoli flowerets	1 cup	120 mL	snow peas	½ cup	120 mL
carrot strips	½ cup				

1. Pour 1 inch (2.54 cm) water into a medium saucepan and add the bay leaf. Boil.
2. Place all vegetables into an expandable steamer basket.
3. Insert the basket into a pot and cover with a tight-fitting lid.
4. Steam the vegetables for approximately 8 to 10 minutes, or until vegetables are tender crisp.
5. Season. (Four to six servings.)

CABBAGE

Remove wilted outside leaves, wash carefully. Cut into wedges or shred. Cook uncovered in water to cover (wedges, 10 to 12 minutes; shredded, 5 to 8 minutes).

Cabbage with Tomato Sauce

green cabbage, shredded	1½ cups	360 mL	tomato sauce	¾	180 mL
onion, minced	¼	60 mL	brown sugar	1 tsp	5 mL
slice bacon, diced (optional)	1				

1. Cook cabbage, uncovered, in water to cover, about 7 minutes. Drain.
2. Sauté onion with bacon (or use 1 tsp [5 mL] oil) until tender.
3. Add tomato sauce and sugar to onion.
4. When sauce comes to a boil, add well-drained cabbage. Season. (Two servings.)

[4] See the chapter on Microwave Cooking for microwave recipes. Season to taste.
[5] See Appendix N, Spice and Herb Chart.
[6] Recipes may contain known allergens. See Appendix E.

Pennsylvania Red Cabbage

vegetable oil	½ tbsp	7.5 mL	water	1 tbsp	15 mL
red cabbage, shredded	1½ cup	360 mL	caraway seed	⅛ tsp	0.63 mL
unpared apple, cubed	½ cup	120 mL	vinegar	½ tbsp	7.5 mL
brown sugar	1 tbsp	15 mL			

1. Heat oil in skillet; add remaining ingredients, except vinegar.
2. Cover tightly; cook over low heat, stirring occasionally.
3. Cook 15 to 25 minutes until desired tenderness is reached.
4. Stir in vinegar. Season. (Two to three servings.)

CARROTS

Scrub. Pare if desired. Leave whole, or cut into crosswise or lengthwise slices. Boil in a small amount of water, covered (10 to 20 minutes).

Glazed Carrots

carrots, medium	3	3	brown sugar	1½ tbsp	22.5 mL
margarine	1½ tbsp	22.5 mL			

1. Cook carrots covered in small amount of boiling water for about 6 to 10 minutes or until tender.
2. In a skillet, melt fat and add brown sugar. Stir until melted.
3. Add the drained carrots and cook slowly, stirring until the carrots are well glazed. Season. (Two servings.)

CAULIFLOWER

1. Remove leaves and some of the woody stem from a quarter of a head of cauliflower. Separate into florets.
2. Cook covered in a small amount of water 10 to 15 minutes or until just tender.
3. Drain and, if desired, add 1 tsp (5 mL) margarine per cup (240 mL) cooked vegetable. Season.

Greek Cauliflower

vegetable oil	1 tbsp	15 mL	canned tomatoes	⅔ cup	160 mL
onion, finely chopped	2 tbsp	30 mL	lemon juice	2 tbsp	30 mL
cauliflower, pieces	2 cup	480 mL	basil	½ tsp	2.5 mL
water	¼ cup	60 mL			

1. In a medium skillet, heat oil. Add onion and sauté until tender.
2. Add cauliflower and water. Cover and cook until just tender.
3. Add chopped tomatoes, lemon juice, and basil to cauliflower.
4. Bring to boil. Reduce heat, cover, and simmer 4 to 6 minutes until flavors blend. Season. (Four servings.)

COLLARDS/KALE

Sautéed Collard Greens/Kale

bacon	1 slice		vegetable oil	1½ tbsp	45 mL
collard greens/kale, fresh	½ lb.	227 g	garlic	1 clove	
water or broth	½ c	120 mL			

1. Fry bacon, drain. Crumble and reserve.
2. Blanch shredded greens for 3 to 5 minutes. Drain.
3. In a medium fry pan, heat oil with garlic for a few minutes. Remove garlic. Add the blanched greens and water. Stir.
4. Cover the pan and cook the greens over low heat for 10 to 15 minutes, stirring occasionally.
5. Drain if necessary. Sprinkle with bacon bits. (Two to three servings.)

EGGPLANT

Baked Eggplant

eggplant, small	1		dry bread crumbs	½ cup	120 mL
evaporated milk	⅓ cup	80 mL	seasonings		

1. Set oven at 400°F (205°C).
2. Peel eggplant and slice ¼ inch (0.63 cm) thick.
3. Dip eggplant into evaporated milk.
4. Combine crumbs and seasonings. Dip eggplant into crumb mixture.
5. Bake on baking sheet 10 to 12 minutes or until tender. Serve with cheese sauce. (Two to three servings.)

Cheese Sauce

Processed cheese	¼ cup	60 mL	evaporated milk	⅓ cup	80 mL

Combine milk and cheese in heavy saucepan or top of double boiler and cook until cheese melts. Stir frequently. If too thick, thin with milk or evaporated milk. Pour over baked eggplant.

Ratatouille (Eggplant–Vegetable Stew)[5]

onion, chopped	¼ cup	60 mL	sliced zucchini	1½ cups	360 mL
green pepper, chopped	½ cup	120 mL	canned tomatoes	¾ cup	180 mL
vegetable oil	2 tbsp	30 mL	tomato sauce	2 tbsp	30 mL
eggplant, diced	2 cups	480 mL	basil, oregano	¼ tsp	1.25 mL

1. In a heavy saucepan or skillet, sauté onion and green pepper in oil until soft.
2. Stir in eggplant and zucchini. Sauté 5 minutes, adding a little more oil, if needed, to prevent sticking.
3. Add tomato, tomato sauce, and seasonings.
4. Cover and boil gently about 25 minutes or until vegetables are tender. Season. (Four to five servings.)

[5] Other vegetables, such as potato, summer squash, mushrooms, and celery, make flavorsome additions.

GREEN BEANS[6]

Wash, remove ends, leave whole or cut crosswise or lengthwise. Boil, uncovered, in small amount of water for a few minutes. Cover and cook until tender. (Whole, 15 to 20 minutes; cut, 8 to 12 minutes.)

Green Beans with Mushrooms (Habichuelas con Hongos)

green beans, sliced	2 cups	480 mL	red pimentos, cut into strips	2	
olive oil	1 tbsp	15 mL	cooked mushrooms, sliced	½ cup	120 mL
onion, minced	2 tbsp	30 mL			

1. Cook green beans, covered, in small amount of water until barely tender.
2. Sauté onion in hot oil. Add cooked beans and pimento. Sauté together for about 5 minutes. Add mushrooms. Heat thoroughly, stirring gently. Season. (Three to four servings.)

ONIONS

Peel under running water. Leave whole, slice, or quarter. Boil in a large amount of water, uncovered. (Slices: 10 minutes; whole 35 minutes.)

Cheese-Scalloped Onions

onion, sliced	1½ cups	360 mL	milk	½ cup	120 mL
margarine	1½ tbsp	22.5 mL	processed cheese	¼ cup	60 mL
all-purpose flour	1½ tbsp	22.5 mL			

1. Set oven at 350°F (175°C).
2. Cook onions uncovered in a large amount of boiling water until nearly tender (6 to 8 minutes); drain well. Place drained onions in a small greased casserole.
3. Melt fat in saucepan, blend in flour.
4. Add milk, cook while stirring until mixture boils.
5. Stir in cheese. Pour sauce over onions.
6. Bake casserole, uncovered about 10 to 15 minutes. Season. (Four servings.)

PLANTAINS

Fried Green Plantains (Tostones)

1. Peel two large green plantains and cut diagonally into slices ½ inch (1.25 cm) thick.
2. Soak slices in a salt solution for about 10 minutes.
3. Dry the slices and fry in vegetable oil at medium heat for about 10 minutes.
4. Remove slices, place on absorbent paper. Fold the paper in half over the slices, and press hard until the slices have been flattened.
5. Refry until golden brown, for about 5 minutes.
6. Remove and drain on absorbent paper to absorb excess oil. Season. Fried plantains may be made ahead and reheated in 400°F (205°C) oven for 5 to 10 minutes. (Note: the recipe may be high in salt.)

---

[6] Beans and peas may be allergenic to some individuals.

POTATOES

Baked Potatoes

1. Set oven at 425°F (220°C).
2. Select smooth potatoes of uniform size. Scrub thoroughly. If soft skin is desired, rub with oil before baking. Prick skin with fork to allow steam to escape.
3. Bake 45 to 60 minutes or until soft.
4. Remove from oven. Serve promptly. If not served immediately, soften potato by rolling in hands, protected with a clean towel.

Stuffed Baked Potatoes

1. Set oven at 425°F (220°C).
2. Cut a slice from the top of an already baked potato or cut in half lengthwise.
3. Scoop out potato pulp, being careful not to break the skin.
4. Mash and season potatoes. (Use 1 to 2 tbsp [15 to 30 mL] milk, 1 tsp [5 mL] margarine.)
5. Pile mixture lightly in the skins, leaving top rough.
6. Place in pan and bake about 10 minutes until delicately browned. Garnish with finely chopped parsley, grated cheese, or paprika.

Stuffed Yams

sweet potato or yam, medium	1		milk	1–2 tbsp	15–30 mL
margarine	1 tbsp	15 mL	chopped walnuts	1 tbsp	15 mL
brown sugar	½ tsp	2.5 mL			

1. Set oven at 400°F (205°C).
2. Scrub potato. Bake 40 minutes or until potato tests done with a fork.
3. Cut potato in half. Scoop out inside, being careful not to break shell.
4. Mash potatoes in a mixing bowl. Add remaining ingredients, except nuts, with enough hot milk to moisten.
5. Beat until fluffy. Fold in nuts. Pile mixture back into potato shell.
6. Bake 15 minutes or until heated through. Season. (One serving.)

SPINACH

Remove root ends and damaged leaves. Break off large stems. If necessary, wash several times until leaves are free of grit and sand. Use only water that clings to the leaves, or a small amount of water. Cook 5 to 7 minutes in a covered pan.

Stir-Fried Spinach

peanut oil	1½ tbsp	22.5 mL	spinach	½ lb.	227 g
clove garlic, crushed	1		water chestnuts	¼ cup	60 mL

1. In a medium frying pan, heat oil with garlic over high heat for a few minutes. Remove garlic.
2. Add spinach and cook, stirring gently approximately 2 minutes until spinach is heated through. Add water chestnuts and season. (Two servings.)

TOMATOES

Baked Tomato

margarine	1 tbsp	15 mL	prepared mustard	½ tsp	2.5 mL
onion, finely chopped	2 tbsp	30 mL	Worcestershire sauce	¼ tsp	1.25 mL
soft bread crumbs	¼ cup	60 mL	tomatoes	2	

1. Set oven at 400°F (205°C).
2. Melt margarine. Add onion and bread crumbs; sauté until onion is soft. Add seasonings.
3. Halve tomato crosswise. Scoop out inside and add to crumb mixture.
4. Fill tomato with mixture. Bake 25 to 30 minutes. Season. (Two servings.)

Mexican Succotash

margarine	1 tbsp	15 mL	corn (fresh, canned, frozen)	½ cup	120 mL
onion, chopped	1 tbsp	15 mL	canned tomatoes	¼ cup	60 mL
zucchini, sliced	1 cup	240 mL			

1. Sauté onion in fat until soft.
2. Add zucchini and corn. Cook covered, 15 minutes or until tender.
3. Add tomatoes; cook just to heat through. Season. (Two servings.)

ZUCCHINI

Zucchini Sauté

1. Wash 1 medium zucchini. Do not pare. Slice thin.
2. Cook, covered, in 1 tbsp (15 mL) margarine in skillet for 5 minutes.
3. Uncover and cook, turning slices until just tender. Season to taste. Sprinkle with 1 tbsp (15 mL) parmesan cheese, if desired. (Two to three servings.)

Zucchini Cheese Casserole

margarine	2 tbsp	30 mL	oregano	¼ tsp	1.25 mL
onion, chopped	¼ cup	60 mL	canned tomatoes	½ cup	120 mL
zucchini, sliced	2 cups	480 mL	processed cheese	¼ cup	60 mL

1. Melt fat in medium frying pan. Add onions, and sauté until tender.
2. Add zucchini and oregano, and cook covered, for 7 minutes or until zucchini is just tender.
3. Add tomatoes, cover and simmer 5 minutes longer. Sprinkle with cheese before serving. Season. (Four servings.)

Stir-Fried Vegetables[7]

oil	2–3 tbsp	30–45 mL	zucchini, sliced	½ cup	120 mL
clove garlic, crushed	1	240 mL	water chestnuts, sliced	¼ cup	60 mL
broccoli, florets	1 cup	120 mL	green pepper, sliced	½ cup	120 mL
carrots, sliced	½ cup	120 mL	snow peas	½ cup	120 mL
summer squash, sliced	½ cup		mung bean sprouts	¼ cup	60 mL

1. Cut vegetables to a similar small size or slice thin.
2. Heat oil in a large skillet or wok, until it is hot, but not smoking. Add garlic.
3. Add broccoli and carrots. Cook 1½ minutes, lifting and turning to expose all sides of the food to the hot pan surface.
4. Add squashes and cook 2 to 3 minutes.
5. Add water chestnuts and cook 1 minute. Cover and let mixture steam 1 to 2 minutes, adding 2 to 3 tbsp (30 to 45 mL) water if dry.
6. Add green pepper, snow peas, and sprouts and cook 1 minute. Sprinkle with soy sauce. (Four to six servings.)

Fat must be extremely hot, but not smoking, for each addition of a new vegetable. Vegetables must be stirred as they are cooked. Vegetables will be done when opaqueness disappears and translucency begins to appear. Vegetables should be crisp, but not taste raw, and hot. Preparation of the vegetables will take the most time, but cooking time is short.

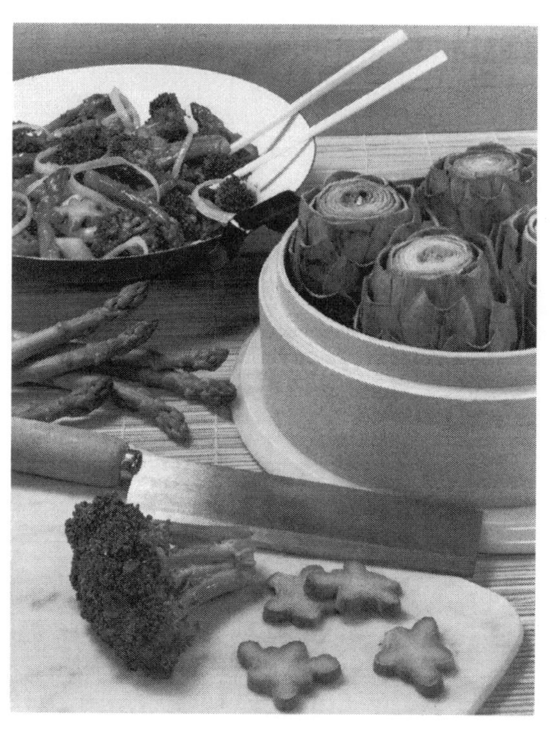

Courtesy: United Fresh Fruit and Vegetable Association.

UNCOOKED VEGETABLES AND FRUIT

Salade Verte–Green Salad

garlic clove, cut	1	1.25 mL	salad oil	2 tbsp	30 mL
salt	¼ tsp	0.60 mL	salad greens, dry, chilled	2 cups	480 mL
dry mustard	¼ tsp	0.60 mL	vinegar	1 tbsp	15 mL
paprika	¼ tsp		lemon juice	1 tbsp	15 mL

1. Rub interior of bowl with cut garlic clove.
2. Combine salt, dry mustard, and paprika with oil.
3. Add mixed greens. Toss in bowl with 1 tbsp vinegar and lemon juice.

Variations: Add 1 cup cooked pasta after step 2. (Two servings.)

[7] Type and amount of vegetables in this recipe may be varied.

Waldorf Salad

red apples, unpared, diced	2 cups	480 mL	walnuts, chopped	½ cup	120 mL
celery, finely diced	¼ cup	180 mL	mayonnaise	to mix	

1. Mix apples, celery, and mayonnaise; sprinkle with nuts.
2. Serve on lettuce leaf. (Six servings.)

RECIPE QUESTIONS—FRUITS AND VEGETABLES

1. Predict the effect on color when milk (pH 6.6) is added to mashed potatoes.

2. Why are cheese-scalloped onions especially mild?

3. Account for the differences in green color observed between zucchini sauté and zucchini casserole.

4. Referring to the glazed carrot recipe, why are the carrots cooked until tender before the sugar is added?

5. In the recipe for Greek cauliflower, why are the tomatoes added after the cauliflower is tender?

SUMMARY QUESTIONS—FRUITS AND VEGETABLES

1. Which vegetables are excellent sources of vitamin A? Vitamin C?

2. As a group, what major nutrients do fruits and vegetable contribute?

3. In addition to vitamins and minerals, what other value do fruits and vegetables have in the daily diet? Which nutrients are most likely to be lost or destroyed during cooking? Indicate what processing factors cause loss.

4. Discuss significant steps in assuring a good color and preventing enzymatic oxidative browning in recipes using cut apples.

5. Based on laboratory experiments, what general principles can be followed to minimize nutrient loss and enhance palatability?

6. Complete the following table with appropriate information for each variable:

Variable	Pigments	Flavors	Nutrients
Water soluble			
Fat soluble			
Volatile			

7. Discuss potential sanitary problems associated with fruits and vegetables. How may these problems be controlled?

8. What storage conditions for vegetables and fruits should be maintained in a grocery store? Why?

9. Provide brief directions for storage of fruits and vegetables in the home.

10. Compare the cost of three fruits and/or vegetables in different forms:

COST COMPARISON

Fruit/Vegetable	Fresh	Frozen	Dried	Canned

Which is the best buy? How would this change with the season? How would this change with intended use?

11. Summarize specific factors that affect cost of fruits and vegetables in the marketplace.

Dietitian's Note

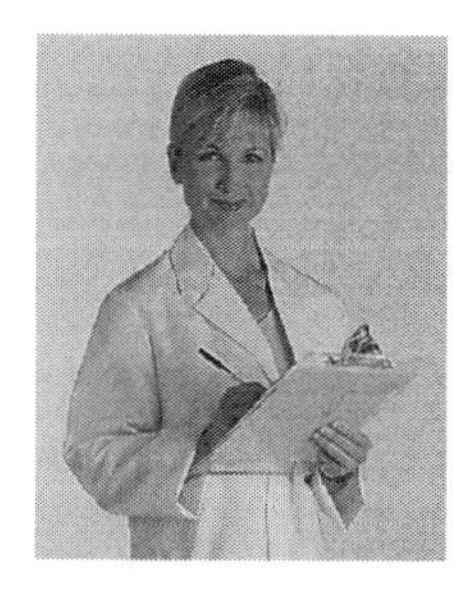

Note on allergens: Vegetable recipes may include a variety of commonly consumed beans and peas. Green beans and peas, not solely legumes such as soybeans and peanuts, may be allergenic to some individuals.

D. Meat, Poultry, and Fish

Fish is brain food. Maybe if you ate some,
you'd understand what I'm talking about!

— Moms everywhere

Objectives

To recognize common retail and prime cuts of meat
To relate location of cut and species to inherent palatability characteristics
To differentiate effects of dry and moist heat on meat products
To demonstrate ability to apply principles of preparation to meat, poultry, and fish
To know and apply principles of sanitary quality to preparation of meat, poultry, and fish
To appraise nutritive and economic dimensions of meat, poultry, and fish products
To identify meat, poultry, and fish allergens and acceptable recipe preparation alternatives

References

Appendices E, H-I, H-II, L-I, L-II, O
www.usda.gov
www.fda.gov
www.beef.org
www.ific.org
http://www.beefitswhatsfordinner.com/recipes/recipe_results.asp
http://www.beef.org/ncbanutrition.aspx Research, Human Nutrition-Vegetarian Diets & Health
http://www.beef.org/uDocs/ACF3A.pdf

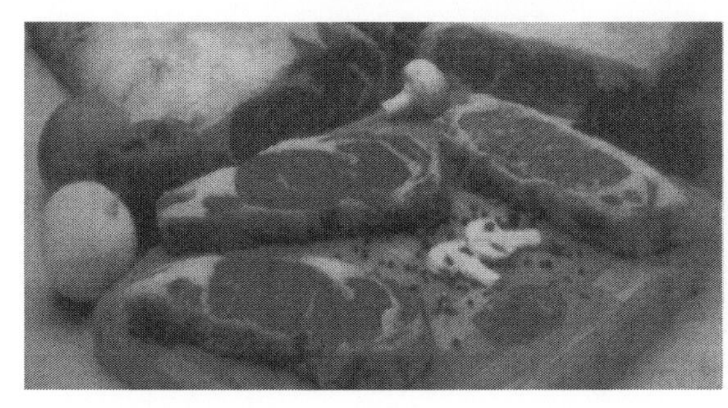

Steak.

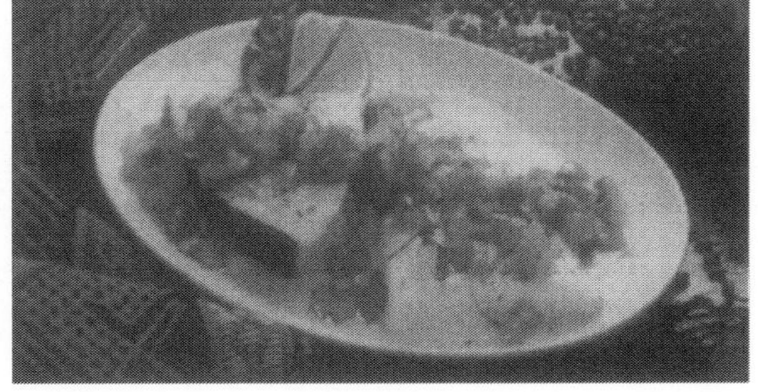

Fish.

Courtesy: SYSCO® Incorporated.

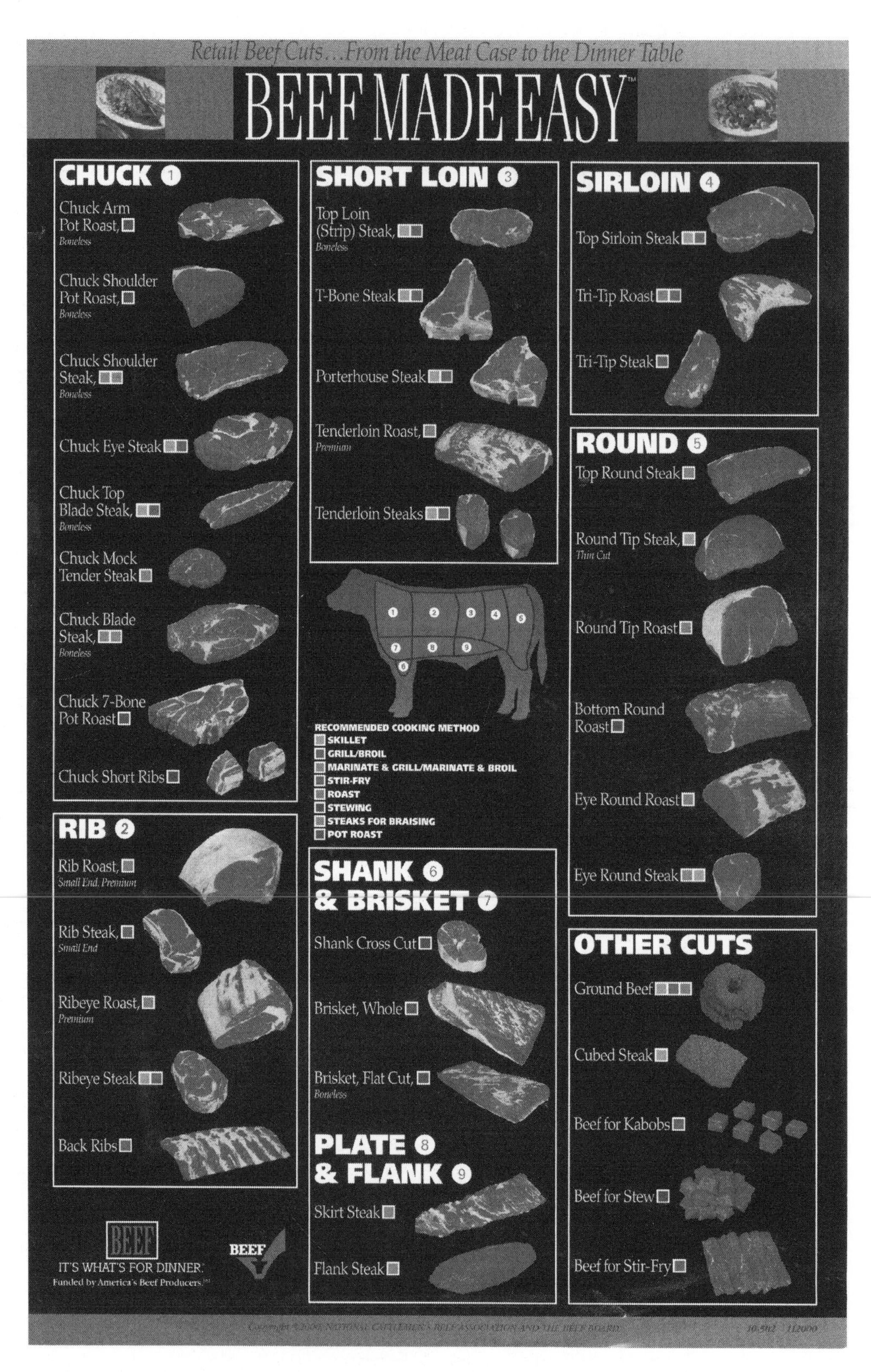

Retail Beef Cuts—Beef Made Easy.

Courtesy: National Cattlemen's Beef Association and The Beef Board.

Terms

Allergens
Bake
Baste
Braise
Bread
Broil, pan broil
Cholesterol
Clostridium perfringens
Collagen
Conformation
Cure
Dry heat cooking
Escherichia coli
Gelatin
Grain
Heart healthy
Inherent tenderness
Marbling
Moist heat cooking
Myosin
Poach
Pot roast
Pressure cook
Roast
Salmonella
Saturated fat
Stew
Stock
Tenderize
Trichinosis
USDA
Wholesomeness

EXERCISE 1: IDENTIFICATION OF BASIC MEAT CUTS

Procedure

1. Study the cuts of meat on display or visit a meat market where various cuts of meat are on display.
2. Complete the following table:

Name of Cut	Prime Cut	Inherent Tenderness	Characteristic Bone, Color, Grain, Marbling	Cost/lb. (454 g)	Cost/ Serving
Beef Blade steak					
Arm steak					
Rib steak					
T-bone or sirloin steak					
Flank steak					
Bottom round					
Top round					
Pork Loin chop					
Rib chop					
Veal Blade steak					
Cutlet					
Lamb Rib chop					
Blade chop					

1. Identify the following markings found on meat and meat products. What do they indicate regarding meat quality and wholesomeness?

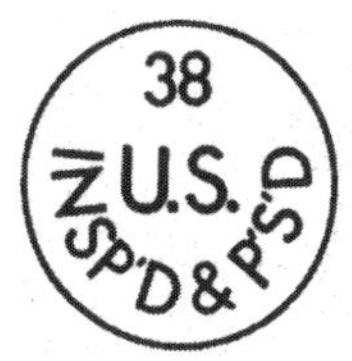

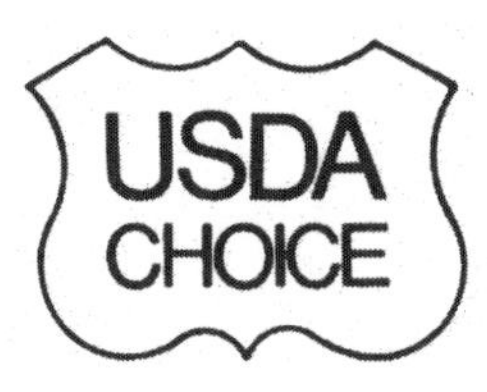

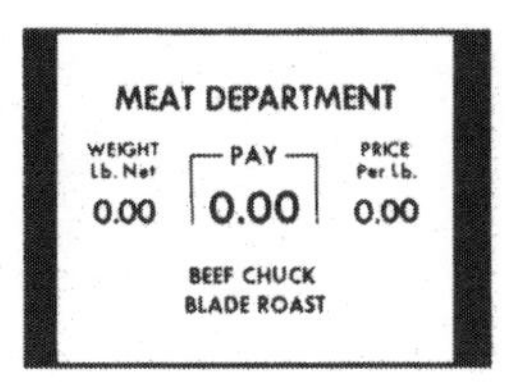

LABELS ON MEAT PRODUCTS.
Courtesy: USDA.

2. What government agency is responsible for inspecting meat and poultry products, both fresh and processed?

3. What generalizations can be made regarding location of a cut of meat and its inherent tenderness?

4. Which is the best way to calculate cost of meat, price per pound or price per serving? Explain.

5. Indicate the approximate number of servings per pound (454 g) of the following products:

beef round:	liver:	spare ribs:
sirloin:	pork chops:	ground chuck:

EXERCISE 2: EFFECT OF DRY AND MOIST HEAT ON LESS TENDER (TOUGH) CUTS OF MEAT

A. Roasts

Procedure

Observe a demonstration prepared as follows:

1. Weigh two roasts (e.g., chuck, bottom round) approximately 2½ lb. (1.14 kg) each (paired cuts if possible). Insert a meat thermometer into each as shown in the photograph.
2. Place one roast uncovered (Roast A) and one roast covered (Roast B) in a 325°F (165°C) oven.
3. Cook roasts until internal temperature of Roast A reaches 77°C (170°F). Record internal temperature of Roast B.
4. Remove both roasts from the oven, weigh, and transfer to serving dish. Record total cooking time.
5. After cooling 10 minutes, slice and evaluate palatability using palatability terms. Summarize results.

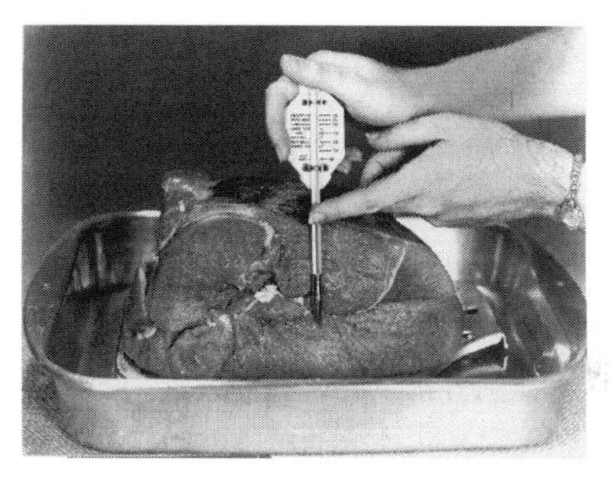

Demonstrating Depth of Meat Thermometer.
Courtesy: USDA.

PALATABILITY TERMS

MOISTNESS	TENDERNESS	FLAVOR
Juicy	Crumbly	Flavorful
Moderately juicy	Tender	Moderately flavorful
Moderately dry	Moderately tender	Moderately bland
Dry	Moderately tough	Bland
	Tough	Tasteless, no flavor

	Roast A—Dry Heat, Uncovered	Roast B—Moist Heat, Covered
Retail cut		
Prime cut		
Inherent tenderness		
Oven temperature	325°F (165°C)	325°F (165°C)
Length of cooking		
Final internal temperature	170°F (77°C)	
Weight loss		
Effect of cooking on muscle fiber		
Effect of cooking on connective tissue		
Moistness		
Tenderness		
Flavor		

1. Relate the observed rate of heat penetration by the dry and moist methods of cooking.

2. Were the roasts equally tender and juicy? Explain.

3. In cooking meat, what is the highest internal temperature obtainable by the moist heat method?

4. Roast A (dry heat) was removed from the oven when the internal temperature reached 170°F (77°C). If the roast were allowed to cook longer, would the internal temperature increase? If so, how would this influence juiciness?

B. Meat Patties[1]

Procedure

1. Prepare two 3-oz. (85-g) patties of ground chuck approximately ½ inch (1.25 cm) thick.
2. Pan-broil one patty, braise the other, following directions specified in the table below.
3. Weigh each patty after cooking and calculate cooking losses.
4. Evaluate both patties, assessing tenderness, juiciness, and flavor.

Pan Broil

1. Place meat in hot, greased pan and cook slowly over moderate heat on one side for 7 minutes.
2. Pour off excess fat as it accumulates.
3. Turn and cook meat for an additional 7 minutes.

Braise

1. Brown meat in 1 tsp (5 mL) oil.
2. Add ⅓ cup (80 mL) hot water to skillet.
3. Cover and simmer for 14 minutes.

	Pan Broiled	Braised
Weight before cooking		
Cooked weight		
Cooking losses		
Tenderness		
Juiciness		
Flavor		

1. How are pan-broiling and braising cooking methods classified? List other examples of the basic methods of cooking meat.

2. Applying principles of protein coagulation, explain the differences in juiciness obtained by the two methods of cooking.

3. What is the effect of grinding (ground beef) on muscle protein? On connective tissue?

[1] If internal temperature of meat patty has not reached 155°F (68°C), do not taste, but observe characteristics of tenderness and juiciness.

4. What techniques, other than grinding, are used to "tenderize" meat? Explain how other techniques work.

EXERCISE 3: EVALUATION OF MEAT, POULTRY, AND FISH

PROCEDURE

1. Inspect a display of meat, poultry, and fish products. Note species' differences in texture, grain, color, and degree of marbling. Consider appearance as related to evidence of freshness.
2. Using assigned recipe, prepare product. Plan cooking so that the product will be hot and ready to serve ____ hours after the start of class.
3. Evaluate all prepared products using terms in this chapter.

Recipe	Appearance Uncooked	Inherent Tenderness	Method of Cooking	Sensory Evaluation	
				Tenderness	Juiciness
Beefsteak					
Beefsteak					
Beefsteak					
Lamb					
Pork					
Veal					
Liver					
Liver					
Liver					
Poultry					
Poultry					
Poultry					
Fish					

(continued on next page)

Recipe	Appearance Uncooked	Inherent Tenderness	Method of Cooking	Sensory Evaluation	
				Tenderness	Juiciness
Fish					
Fish					
Fish					
Shrimp					
Scallops					

MEAT, POULTRY, AND FISH RECIPES[2,3]

BEEF

Broiled Steak (Sirloin, T-bone, Rib, Porterhouse Steak)

1. Grease broiler rack and preheat broiler. (Follow oven directions on use of broiler.)
2. Slash the outer fat of the meat in several places to prevent curling.
3. After allowing meat to stand at room temperature for a few minutes, place meat on broiler rack.
4. Broil 3 to 4 inches (7.5 to 10 cm) from heat. Rate of heat is regulated by distance meat is placed from heating unit.
5. Turn steak when upper side is brown. Season to taste.

Broiled Flank Steak—London Broil

1. Grease broiler rack and preheat broiler.
2. Allow meat to stand a few minutes at room temperature. Score meat by cutting diagonally across the long muscle fibers.
3. Place steak on rack. Broil 2 to 3 inches (5 to 7.5 cm) from heat about 5 minutes on each side. Cook to rare. Carve across grain.

Pan-Broiled Steak

1. Slash the outer fat edge in several places to prevent curling.
2. Place meat in heavy frying pan.
3. Cook, uncovered, slowly. Do not add fat or water. (Pour fat from pan as it accumulates.)
4. Turn meat to brown the other side. Cook to desired doneness. Season.

[2] Review information in Appendix G-II concerning regulations about cooking temperatures for meat and poultry.
[3] Recipes may contain known allergens. See Appendix E.

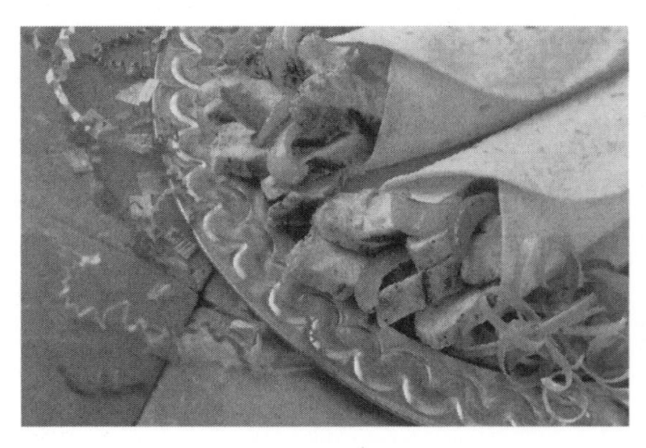

Chicken Fajitas.

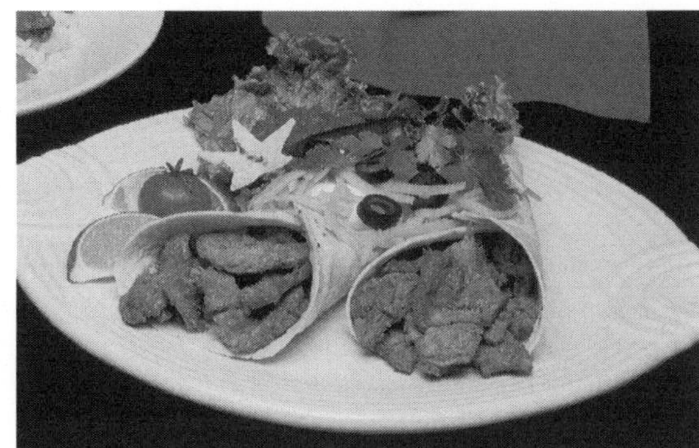

Beef Fajitas.

Courtesy: SYSCO® Incorporated.

Beef Fajitas[4]

1. Sauté an onion and a green pepper in 2 teaspoons of oil.
2. Add sliced beef or a 6-oz. package of prepared seasoned beef slices (or chicken).
3. Heat through and wrap in tortillas[5] to serve. Top as desired prior to wrapping—with salsa, sour cream, lime juice, etc.

Meatballs[4]

1. Heat prepared meatballs in spaghetti sauce.
2. Use meatballs to top spaghetti; or
3. Place in a sub (hero/hoagie/wedge/poorboy)-type roll, top with mozzarella cheese, and broil.

LAMB

Curry of Lamb

lamb (round)	⅓ lb.	151 g	chopped green pepper	¼ cup	60 mL
margarine	2 tbsp	30 mL	curry powder	1–2 tsp	5–10 mL
clove of garlic	1		apple, diced	½	
finely chopped onion	½ cup	120 mL	carrot, diced	½	
chopped celery	¼ cup	60 mL			

1. Cut meat into 1- to 2-inch (2.5- to 5-cm) pieces, and brown lightly in fat.
2. Push meat to one side of frying pan. Add garlic, onion, celery, and green pepper to pan, and cook slowly for 2 to 3 minutes. Remove garlic.
3. Add remaining ingredients, and mix with meat.
4. Cover and simmer in water until meat is tender, about 1 hour.

Note: Cooked lamb, beef, chicken, or fish may be used. (Two servings.)

---

[4] Quick to fix.

[5] Typically contains gluten.

PORK

Pan-Broiled Pork Chops

1. Place two pork chops in heavy frying pan.
2. Over moderate heat, brown each side of the chops.
3. Reduce heat. Cook chops slowly, uncovered.
4. Pour off excess grease as it accumulates.
5. Cook until chops are well done. Season. (Two servings.)

Braised Pork Chops

pork chops	2		chili powder	¼ tsp	1.25 mL
oil	1 tbsp	15 mL	chopped onion	1 tbsp	15 mL
tomato sauce	½ cup	120 mL	vinegar	1½ tbsp	22.5 mL
Worcestershire sauce	1 tsp	5 mL			

1. Brown chops in oil. Pour off excess fat.
2. Combine remaining ingredients. Add to chops.
3. Cook, covered, 25 to 30 minutes, or until chops are done. (Two servings.)

VEAL

Breaded Veal Cutlet

veal cutlets	2		egg, slightly beaten	1	
flour* to coat			fine bread crumbs	⅓ cup	80 mL
oregano			oil	1–2 tbsp	15–30 mL

* Typically contains gluten.

1. Dip veal cutlet in seasoned flour.
2. Dip cutlet into egg, then in crumbs. Let dry 5 minutes.
3. Pan-fry slowly in hot oil in heavy skillet (about 15 minutes each side). Serve as is, or with a tomato sauce. (Two servings.)

LIVER

Chopped Chicken Livers

egg	1		oil	1 tbsp	15 mL
chicken livers	⅓ lb.	454 g	mayonnaise	2 tbsp	30 ml
finely chopped onion	¼ cup	60 mL			

1. Simmer egg until hard. Cool, shell.
2. Simmer chicken livers until just tender. Drain and cool.
3. Sauté onion in oil. Add to liver and egg. Chop and mix until livers are a fine paste or force through a food grinder. Add mayonnaise, mix, and season. Chill and serve with crackers.

Crisp Liver Strips

beef liver	⅓ lb.	454 g	egg, slightly beaten	1	120 mL
fat-free French dressing	¼ cup	60 mL	cracker crumbs*	½ cup	30–45 mL
			vegetable oil	2–3 tbsp	

* Typically contains gluten.

1. Cut liver into ½-inch (1.25-cm) strips.
2. Marinate in dressing 5 to 10 minutes. Drain.
3. Dip in beaten egg. Roll in cracker crumbs. Let dry 5 minutes.
4. Fry in hot fat. Drain, season, and serve. (Two to three servings.)

Pan-Fried Liver

beef liver	½ lb	227 g	oil	2 tbsp	30 mL
green pepper, cut into strips	¼		stewed tomatoes	¾ cup	180 mL
onion, sliced	1				

1. Cut liver into pieces.
2. Sauté liver, green pepper, and onion in oil until liver is lightly brown.
3. Add tomatoes and simmer 10 minutes until just tender. Season. If desired, thicken gravy with ½ tbsp (7.5 mL) flour. (Two to three servings.)

POULTRY

Chicken Cacciatore

chopped onion	⅓ cup	80 mL	garlic clove	1	
boiling water	¼ cup	60 mL	oregano	½ tsp	2.5 mL
canned tomatoes	1 cup	240 mL	olive slices	2 tbsp	30 mL
tomato puree	¼ cup	60 mL	chicken breast halves	2	

1. Cook onion in boiling water. Do not drain.
2. Add all ingredients, except chicken. Simmer 10 minutes to blend flavors.
3. Place breast halves in heavy frying pan. Pour tomato mixture over chicken.
4. Cook, covered, over low heat until chicken is tender, about 30 to 35 minutes. (Two servings.)

Oven-Fried Chicken

chicken, cut into pieces	half		garlic powder	dash	
oil or Italian dressing	2–3 tbsp	30–45 mL			

1. Set oven at 375°F (190°C).
2. Place chicken, skin side up (or use skinless) in baking pan to which oil or dressing has been added.
3. Turn chicken to coat with oil, cook skin side down. Season.
4. Bake 40 minutes uncovered. If desired, turn chicken in the last 10 minutes to brown all sides. (Two servings.)

Stir-Fried Chicken

chicken breast, sliced	1	5 mL	chicken broth	1 cup	240 mL
peanut oil	1 tsp	60 mL	low-sodium soy sauce	2 tbsp	30 mL
green pepper, sliced	¼ cup	60 mL	green onion	2	10 mL
chopped onion	¼ cup	120 mL	cold water	2 tsp	10 mL
broccoli florets	½ cup	120 mL	cornstarch	2 tsp	480 mL
sliced mushrooms	½ cup		cooked rice	2 cups	

1. Cook chicken in oil by rapidly lifting and turning the sliced pieces to expose all of the raw surfaces to the hot pan surface. Remove from skillet or push up sides of pan or wok.
2. Cook pepper and onion in skillet for a few minutes, turning constantly.
3. Add broccoli, mushrooms, broth, and soy sauce, cooking 5 minutes.
4. Add chicken back to mixture, cooking 2 to 3 minutes, keeping vegetables tender crisp. Add onion.
5. Mix cornstarch with cold water, stir into hot mixture, and cook just to thicken.
6. Remove from heat and serve with hot rice. (Two servings.)

Chicken and Greens Salad[6]

1. Portion a ready-to-eat, bagged salad of mixed greens into 4 bowls.
2. Top each of the bowls evenly with 3 oz. of cooked chicken (or packaged, prepared chicken cubes) and 2 tablespoons (30 mL) Italian salad dressing.

FISH[7]

Broiled Fish

fish fillets	½ lb	227 g	low-fat Italian salad dressing	¼ cup	60 mL

1. Turn on broiler.
2. Brush fish with dressing.
3. Place on preheated, greased broiler rack, skin side down, about 2 inches (5 cm) from the heat.
4. Broil until browned, turn with a wide spatula turner, and brown the other side.
5. Baste with dressing if dry. Broil 10 minutes or until fish flakes. Season. (Two to three servings)

Fish Chowder

fish	⅓ lb	151 g	potatoes, diced	½ cup	120 mL
water	1½ cup	360 ml	milk	1 cup	240 mL
fat salt pork, diced (or oil)	1 tbsp	15 mL	evaporated milk	½ cup	120 mL
chopped onions	¼ cup	60 mL			

1. Clean the fish. Poach fish by placing in water. Simmer, covered, until fish flakes.
2. Meanwhile, cook salt pork in a skillet until golden brown and crisp, remove, and drain almost all fat; add onion and cook until soft (or sauté onion in oil).

[6] Quick to fix.
[7] Haddock, perch, sole, flounder, turbot, or cod are suggested.

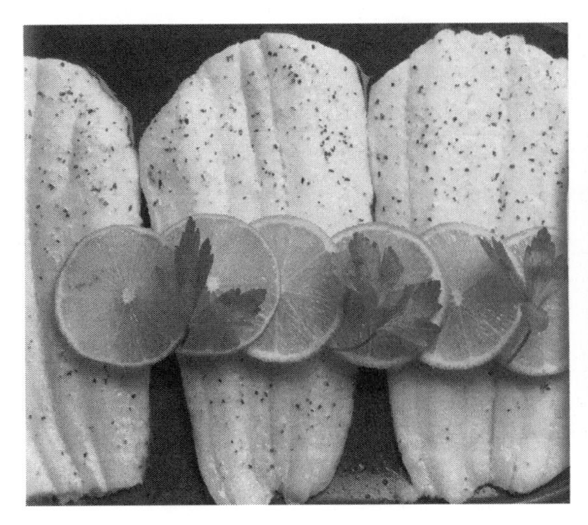
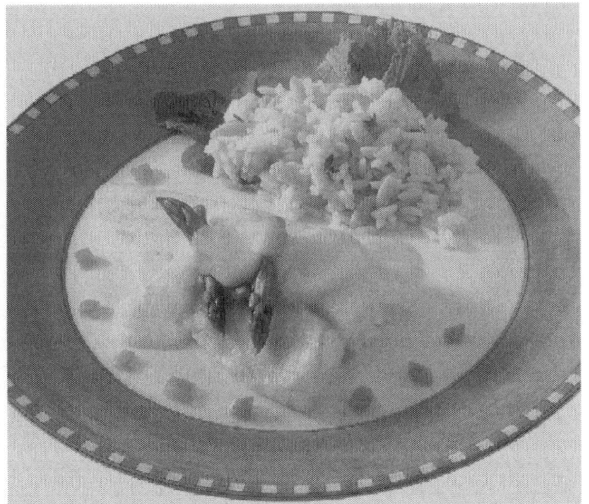

FISH.
Courtesy: SYSCO® Incorporated.

3. Remove cooked fish from water; pour ½ cup (120 mL) of cooking water over the onions, add the diced potatoes, and cook until tender, about 10 minutes. Add both types of milk.
4. Separate fish carefully into flakes and add to milk, potatoes, and onions. Simmer to reheat fish. Season and, if desired, add salt pork.

Quick Oven-Baked Fish

fish fillets	½ lb.	227 g	fine bread/cornflake crumbs	½ cup	120 mL
milk (whole or evaporated)	¼ cup	60 mL	margarine	1 tbsp	15 mL

1. Set oven at 500°F (260°C).
2. Dip fillets in milk. Roll in crumbs.
3. Place fish skin-side down in a greased baking pan.
4. Drizzle with melted fat.
5. Bake 7 to 10 minutes (or until fish flakes, depending upon the thickness). Season. (Two servings.)

Spicy Baked Fish

fish fillets or swordfish	½ lb.	227 g	oil	2 tsp	10 mL
chopped onion	¼ cup	60 mL	canned tomatoes	1 cup	240 mL
chopped green pepper	¼ cup	60 mL			

1. Set oven at 350°F (175°C).
2. Cut fish into two servings. Place in greased baking dish.
3. Bake until fish flakes easily, about 20 minutes. Drain liquid from fish.
4. Meanwhile, cook onion and pepper in oil until clear.
5. Cut up large pieces of tomatoes. Add tomatoes. Cook to blend flavors.
6. Pour sauce over drained fish. Bake at 350°F (175°C) for 7 to 10 minutes. Season. (Two servings.)

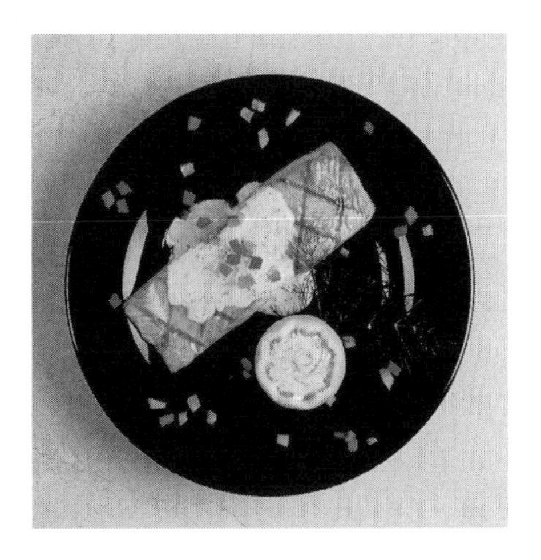

SALMON.
Courtesy: SYSCO® Incorporated.

Salmon Noodle Salad[8]

salmon, rectangular cuts	⅓ lb	151 g	vinaigrette dressing	¼ cup	60 mL
fettuccine noodles, cooked*	2 cups	480 mL	(if served cold)		

* Typically contains gluten.

1. Broil salmon 5 to 10 minutes until it flakes and is done.
2. Serve hot or place cooked portion of cold salmon atop cooked, chilled noodles. Add dressing. (Two servings.)

SHELLFISH

Simmered Shrimp

water	1 cup	240 mL	sprig parsley	1	5 mL
peppercorns	4		vinegar	1 tsp	227 g
bay leaf	1		shrimp	½ lb.	
stalk celery	½				

1. Simmer the water with all ingredients except the shrimp for about 5 minutes.
2. Remove the shells from shrimp. With a knife, cut the shrimp just below the surface down the back. Lift out the black sand vein.
3. Add the shrimp to the stock. Cover the pan and simmer the shrimp for 5 minutes. Do not boil. Drain and chill the shrimp. Season with cocktail sauce or add to a curry or Creole sauce.

Cocktail Sauce: Blend and chill: ¼ cup (60 mL) tomato sauce, ¼ cup (60 mL) chili sauce, 1 tbsp (15 mL) grated horseradish, squeeze of fresh lemon
Or ketchup with squeeze of one fresh lemon.
Yield: ½ cup (120 mL).

[8] Quick to fix.

Baked Scallops and Bacon

slices bacon	3	scallops	⅓ lb	151 g

1. Precook bacon until lightly brown. Remove from heat, drain, cut into 2-inch (5-cm) pieces, reserve fat.
2. Wash scallops to remove all sand. If scallops are large, cut them in half.
3. Cook scallops for 2 to 3 minutes in 2 tbsp (30 mL) reserved bacon fat.
4. Wrap bacon pieces around scallops and place on skewers. Place skewers across baking dish.
5. Bake at 350°F (175°C) until bacon is crisp, 10 to 12 minutes. (Two servings.)

SUMMARY QUESTIONS—MEAT, POULTRY, AND FISH

1. Make a summary statement concerning the relationship of the inherent tenderness of a cut of meat and its price. Discuss whether a similar generalization can be applied to the comparison of a cut of meat and its nutritive value.

2. List four "dry-heat" methods of cooking.

3. List four "moist-heat" methods of cooking.

4. List cuts of meat that are often breaded. What method of cooking is used for breaded products?

5. Predict the outcome as to relative juiciness and tenderness, if a pressure cooker was used to stew a bottom round. Explain.

6. Select an appropriate method of cooking for each of the following products. Explain.

Product	Method	Explanation
Heart		
Liver		
Cod fillets		
Shrimp		
Fowl (mature hen)		

7. Based on laboratory observations and/or readings, discuss internal cooking temperatures of meat in relation to palatability characteristics of a meat product.

Degree of Doneness	Internal Temperature	Palatability
Rare		
Medium		
Well done		

8. Complete the following nutritive value chart.

Food Item, 3 oz. (90 g)	Energy (kcal)	Protein (g)	Fat (g)	Cholesterol (mg)	Iron (g)
Beef liver					
Ground beef					
Chicken breast					
Haddock					
Pork chop					
Veal					

9. In summary, identify the major nutrient contributions of meat, poultry, and fish.

10. Which nutrients in meats are adversely affected by long cooking time or high cooking temperatures?

11. Ground turkey may be substituted for beef in ground meat recipes, or it may be processed into lunchmeat and hot dogs. What are the advantages of using turkey meat?

12. When a large roast is removed from the oven, what happens to the internal temperature? Explain. Based on this fact, how can a roast be cooked to only the medium-done stage?

13. Recipes for roasting turkey over 15 pounds (6.8 kg) include directions to bake stuffing separately. Why is separate roasting necessary?

14. Complete the following chart (see Appendix H-II).

Meat	End Cooking Temperature	Microorganism Needing Control
Beef		
Pork		
Chicken		
Ground beef patty		

15. Why does ground beef have a shorter shelf life than the roast from which it came? What other flesh products are considered highly perishable?

16. List several precautions that should be taken in the use of cutting boards and knives that have been used to cut items such as chicken, beef, pork, or fish.

17. Apply principles of time and temperature interaction to the preservation of the sanitary quality of meat.

18. Explain why "Quick Oven-Baked Fish" is tender and juicy, yet the 500°F (260°C) oven temperature appears to contradict the principle of using low temperatures for protein foods.

19. At current prices, which of the following would be the best protein buy per serving: beef liver? hot dogs? hamburger? haddock?

20. Identify "Safe Handling Instructions" that appear on meat packages.

21. Relate the graph shown below to the cooking of an inherently tough and an inherently tender cut of meat:

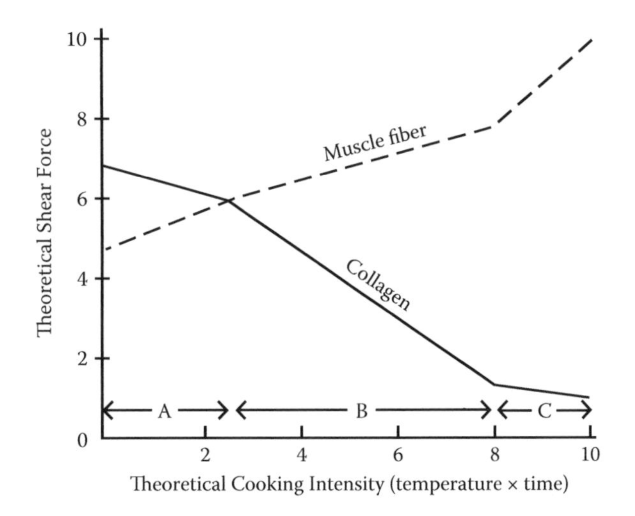

Source: Wang, H.H. et al. 1954. Food Research® Institute of Food Technologists, Chicago, IL. With permission.

a. According to theoretical cooking intensity shown in the graph, for which cut would an increasingly "tough, dry" product be expected over time? Explain.

b. For which cut would greater cooking intensity be advantageous? Explain.

c. Select one recipe from the meat unit and explain how cooking intensity (time and temperature) was used to achieve a palatable product.

22. Identify generalizations that may be made concerning the use of a crock pot for cooking meats or poultry with regard to cut of meat, tenderness, and cooking time.

23. How are meat, poultry, or fish products implicated in food allergies?

Dietitian's Note

Heart Healthy Eating: Choose lean, low-fat, low-salt, appropriate portion sizes. See websites:

http://www.healthierus.gov/dietaryguidelines/index.html
www.mypyramid.gov
www.nal.usda.gov/fnic/etext/000036.html
http://ars.usda.gov - browse nutrition
http://www.mypyramid.gov/guidelines/index.html

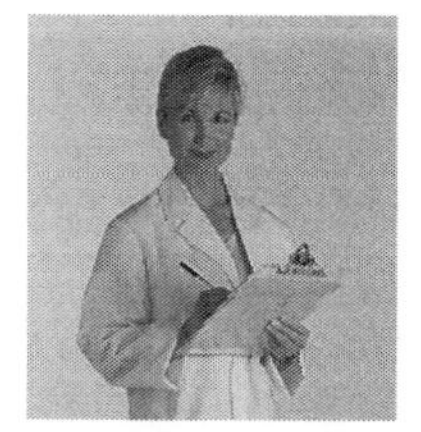

The **Dietary Guidelines for Americans**, 2005 (U.S. Department of Health and Human Services and USDA), gives science-based advice on food and physical activity choices for health. See the full 80-page *Dietary Guidelines* report.

What is a "healthy diet"?

The *Dietary Guidelines* describe a **healthy diet** as one that:

- Emphasizes fruits, vegetables, whole grains, and fat-free or low-fat milk and milk products;
- Includes lean meats, poultry, fish, beans, eggs, and nuts; and
- Is low in saturated fats, trans fats, cholesterol, salt (sodium), and added sugars.

The recommendations in the Dietary Guidelines and in MyPyramid are for the general public over 2 years of age. MyPyramid is not a therapeutic diet for any specific health condition. Individuals with a chronic health condition should consult with a health care provider to determine what dietary pattern is appropriate for them.

Allergens: Read labels! Allergens that appear in meat and fish recipes may include milk, eggs, wheat (breading, thickeners), soybean ingredients, and so forth. Vinegar may be made from wheat. Soy sauce may contain wheat!

E. Plant Proteins

To make good soup, the pot must only simmer or smile.

— French proverb

Objectives

To demonstrate how to rehydrate and cook legumes and to understand principles involved in achieving a palatable product

To identify the nutritive value of combinations of grains, legumes, and seeds as meat alternatives

To identify various combinations of grains, legumes, and seeds, as well as combinations with milk, which provide a complete amino acid pattern

To become familiar with a variety of meat alternatives by incorporating them into palatable, nutritious recipes

To appraise the nutritive, sanitary, and economic dimensions of plant proteins

To identify plant protein foods with known allergens

References

Appendices E, N, O

Gollman, B. and K. Pierce. 1998. *The Phytopia Cookbook: A World of Plant-Centered Cuisine*. Dallas, TX: Phytopia, Inc.

www.phytopia.com

Terms

Allergen
Complete protein
Essential amino acid
Incomplete protein
Lacto-ovo vegetarian
Legumes
Lentils
Lysine
Mutual supplementation
Partially complete protein
Pectin
PER
Sulfur-containing amino acids
Tryptophan
Vegetarian vegan

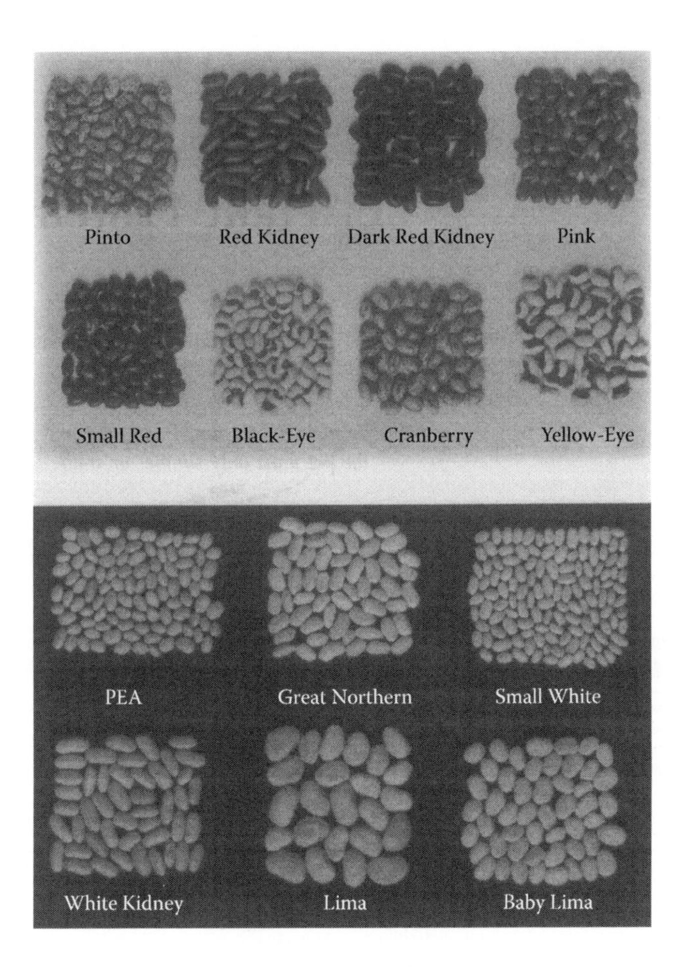

Principal Types of Beans.
(Top) Dry, Colored Beans; (Bottom) Dry, White Beans.
Courtesy: USDA.

Exercise 1: Pretreatment and Cooking Methods for Legumes[1]

A. Pretreatment

Procedures (1 or 2)

1. Add 1½ cups (360 mL) water to ½ cup (120 mL) assigned beans. Bring to a boil and boil 2 to 3 minutes. Turn off heat and soak, covered, for 1 hour.
2. Add 1½ cups (360 mL) water to assigned beans, cover, refrigerate overnight. (The longer the beans are soaked, the less gas-producing they will be. Drain the soaking water.)

[1] Legumes = pulses. Notes: Legumes are plants that have pods with tidy rows of seeds inside. This category includes beans, peas, lentils, and peanuts. (The Cook's Thesaurus)

B. Cooking Methods

Beans: Place pretreated beans in uncovered saucepan, adding water to cover if necessary, and boil. Lower heat and simmer until beans are tender. A slow cooker with several inches of water covering the beans may be used as the cooking method. This takes 4 or more hours on low. Additional water may be necessary.

Lentils/split peas: Place ½ cup (120 mL) unsoaked lentils or split peas in saucepan and cover with water. Cook until tender. A slow cooker as noted above for beans may be used to produce acceptable lentils or split peas. Cooking time may be 3 or more hours on low.

Procedure

Record time and cooked yield. If using in Exercise 2, place in covered containers, refrigerate, or freeze.

	Cooking Time	Cooked Yield	Palatability (your own ideas)
Black beans			
Black-eyed peas			
Garbanzo beans (chickpeas)			
Great northern beans			
Lentils			
Lima beans			
Navy beans			
Red kidney beans			
Soybeans			
Split peas			
Other:			

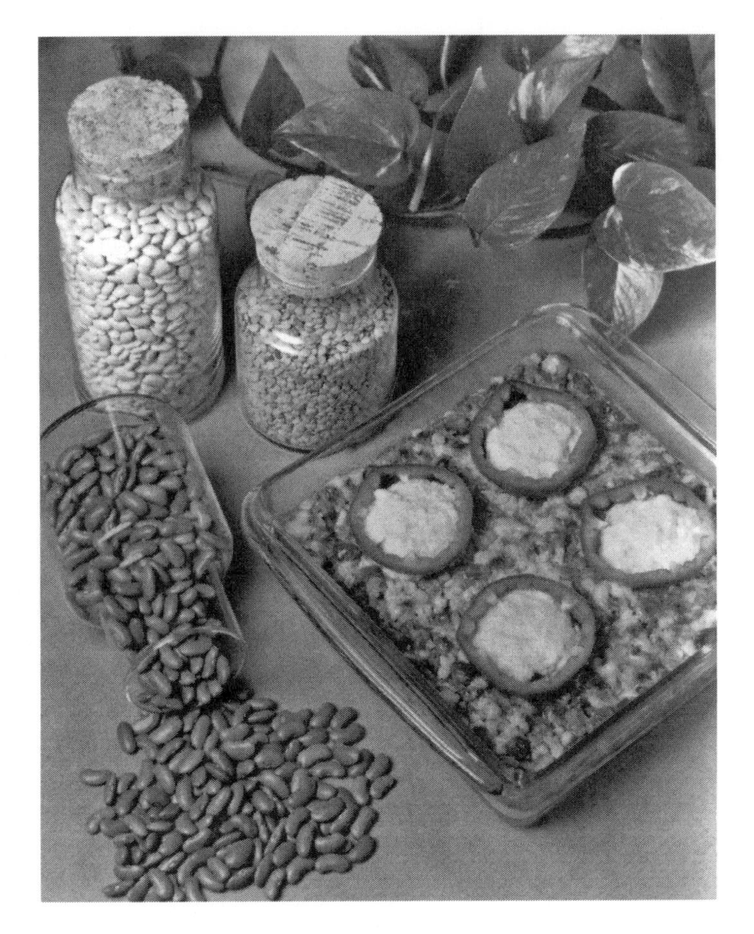

Vegetable Protein Casserole.

Source: Division of Nutritional Sciences, New York State College of Human Ecology at Cornell, Ithaca, New York.

EXERCISE 2: COMBINING PLANT PROTEINS

Procedure

1. Follow directions for assigned product. Plan to serve in an hour.
2. Display product and evaluate all finished products for palatability, nutritive value, and general acceptability. (For recipes calling for cooked beans, a crock pot may be used for cooking the beans if time permits.)

Note: Peanuts are a PEA, NOT a nut.

EVALUATION OF PLANT PROTEIN RECIPES

Recipe	Plant Protein	Palatability			Comments
		Appearance	Texture	Flavor	

PLANT PROTEIN RECIPES[2,3]

Frijoles (Beans)

cooked red or pinto beans	2½ cups	600 mL	cooked tomatoes	1 cup	120 mL
chili powder	½ tsp	2.5 mL	chopped celery	⅓ cup	60 mL
cayenne pepper	⅛ tsp	0.63 mL	cooked rice	2 cups	480 mL
chopped onion	⅓ cup	80 mL			

1. Combine all ingredients except rice and simmer, covered, about 30 minutes. Stir occasionally. Season.
2. Serve over rice. (Two to three servings.)

Beans and Rice Casserole

beans, cooked (garbanzo, red	2¼ cups	660 mL	green pepper, chopped	¼ cup	60 mL
beans, pinto beans, etc.)		7.5 mL	garlic clove, chopped	2	
oil	½ tbsp	60 mL	tomato sauce	¾ cup	180 mL
finely chopped onion	¼ cup	120 mL	basil	½ tsp	2.5 mL
finely chopped carrots	2		oregano	½ tsp	2.5 mL
chopped celery	½ cup		cooked rice	1 cup	240 mL
			grated cheese	2–3 tbsp	30–45 mL

1. In a large skillet, sauté onion, carrots, celery, pepper, and garlic in oil until softened.
2. Add beans, tomato sauce, and seasonings; simmer 15 minutes.
3. Combine rice and bean mixture, or spoon bean mixture over rice. Sprinkle with cheese. (Two to three servings.)

Variation: May be cooked with ground meat, without rice, and served with fresh tomatoes and salsa over tossed greens in a taco shell.

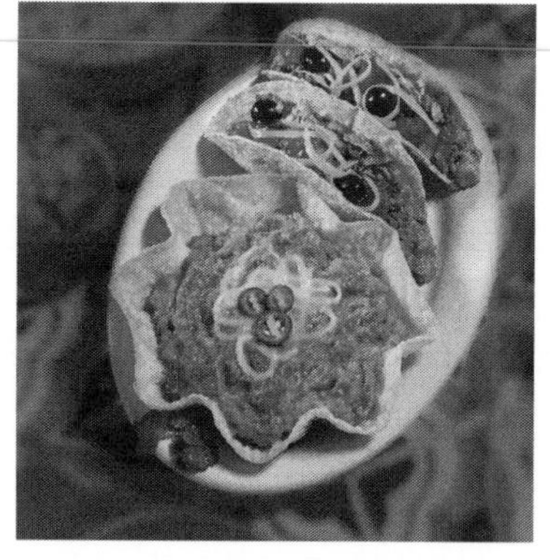

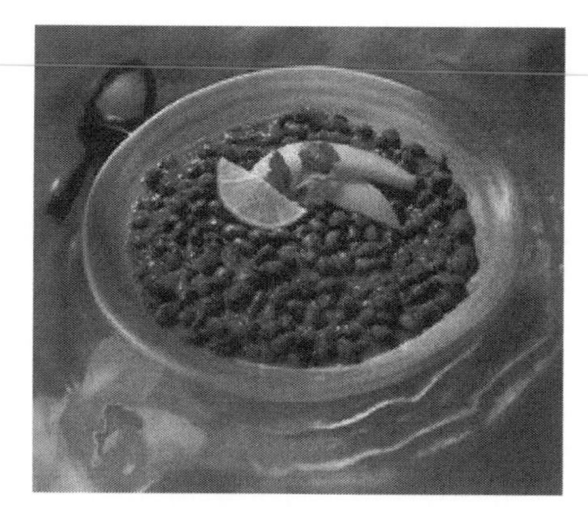

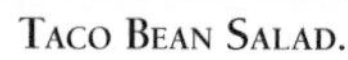

Taco Bean Salad.

Black Bean Soup.

Courtesy: SYSCO® Incorporated.

[2] Cooked (canned) beans are used to conserve preparation time. Therefore, drain and wash to reduce salt.
[3] Recipes may contain known allergens. See Appendix E.

Many Bean Soup

chopped celery	½ cup	120 mL	liquid* from beans or water	1 cup	240 mL
chopped onion	⅓ cup	80 mL	cooked beans (navy, kidney, lima, etc.)	2 cups	480 mL
oil	1 tbsp	15 mL	cooked tomatoes, mashed	½ cup	120 mL
sliced carrots	1 cup	240 mL	dill weed	½ tsp	2.5 mL
medium potato, diced	1				

* Add liquid until desired consistency is achieved.

1. In a medium saucepan, sauté celery and onion in oil until soft.
2. Add carrots, potatoes, and liquid. Boil until vegetables are just tender.
3. Add beans, tomatoes, and dill weed. Simmer gently until mixture is heated through. Season. Serve with a grain product. (Four servings.)

Black Bean Soup with Onion and Herbs

olive oil	1 tbsp	15 mL	black beans, canned, undrained	15.5 oz. cans	2 cans
chopped onion	1		water	2 cups	480 mL
garlic clove, chopped	1		red pepper flakes	½ tsp	2.5 mL
ground cumin	1 tsp	5 mL	bay leaf	1	
dried oregano	1 tsp	5 mL	salt and pepper	½ tsp	2.5 mL

1. In a heavy pan sauté onion for 4 minutes. Add garlic, cumin, and oregano and sauté 1 minute.
2. Add undrained beans, water, pepper flakes, and bay leaf, bringing to a boil. Reduce heat, simmering uncovered for 20 minutes.
3. Season with salt and pepper and cook 5 minutes.
4. Garnish with cilantro leaf. (Four servings.)

Cornmeal–Bean Bread

oil	1 tbsp	15 mL	stock from beans (or beef bouillon)	1¼ cups	300 mL
chopped onion	¼ cup	60 mL	egg, beaten	1	
cornmeal	1 cup	240 mL	grated cheese	¼ cup	60 mL
baking powder	2 tsp	10 mL	sliced black olives	¼ cup	60 mL
chili powder	½ tbsp	7.5 mL			
cooked kidney beans, chopped	1½ cups	360 mL			

1. Set oven at 350°F (175°C).
2. Sauté onion in oil in medium skillet. Remove onion and reserve.
3. Mix cornmeal, baking powder, and seasonings in a bowl.
4. Combine onion, kidney beans, stock, and egg. Add to dry ingredients, mixing just to moisten.
5. Pour mixture into skillet. Sprinkle with cheese and olives. Season.
6. Bake 15 minutes or until bread tests done. (Four servings.)

Eggplant Casserole

cooked tomatoes, drained	1 cup	240 mL	sesame seed	¼ cup	60 mL
oregano	½ tsp	2.5 mL	large eggplant, peeled, sliced	½	
thyme	¼ tsp	1.25 mL	oil	2 tsp	10 mL
finely chopped onion	2 tbsp	30 mL	mozzarella cheese, sliced	¼ lb	114 g
chopped green pepper	2 tbsp	30 mL	cooked rice	1½ cups	360 mL
grated cheese (parmesan or cheddar)	¼ cup	60 mL			

1. Set oven at 350°F (175°C).
2. Combine tomatoes, seasonings, onion, and green pepper. Cover and simmer 10 to 15 minutes. Add grated cheese and sesame seed.
3. Meanwhile, using a large frying pan, sauté eggplant slices in oil until lightly browned. Drain.
4. Place a layer of eggplant in a 2-quart (2-L) greased baking dish. Cover with half the tomato sauce and half the mozzarella cheese. Repeat layers.
5. Bake about 30 minutes until cheese browns. Serve with rice. Season. (Three servings.)

Enchiladas–Bean and Cheese

vegetable oil	3 tbsp	45 mL	water	3 cups	720 mL
flour	3 tbsp	45 mL	refried beans	1½ cups	360 mL
chili powder	3 tbsp	45 mL	corn tortillas	12	
tomato bouillon with chicken flavor	1 tbsp	15 mL	jack cheese	½ cup	120 mL

1. Brown flour. Add chili powder and oil.
2. Add water and bouillon. Stir. Bring to a boil until sauce thickens, stirring well.
3. Dip tortillas into sauce. Fill each tortilla with 1 tbsp (15 mL) heated refried beans and roll up tortilla.
4. Arrange in a casserole dish and pour remaining sauce on top. Sprinkle with cheese.
5. Place in 350°F (175°C) oven 10 to 15 minutes to melt cheese.

Variation: Use beans in place of meat in beef tacos.

Hoppin' John

bacon, slice	1		cooked black beans	1 cup	240 mL
finely chopped onion	¼ cup	60 mL	cooked rice	1 cup	240 mL
garlic clove, minced (optional)	1		water or chicken stock	⅓ cup	80 mL

1. Fry bacon, onion, and garlic in saucepan. Remove bacon when crisp, drain, and crumble. Reserve.
2. Add beans, rice, and water to fat.
3. Bring to boil, lower heat, and simmer 10 minutes. Season and add bacon. (Two to three servings.)

Hummus (Garbanzo–Tahini Spread) with Pita Bread

onion, minced	1 large		lemon juice, fresh	½ cup	120 mL
garlic, minced clove	1		soy sauce, reduced-sodium	1 tbsp	15 mL
oil, vegetable	1 tbsp	15 mL	sesame paste (tahini)	¼ cup	60 mL
garbanzo beans	2 cups	480 mL	pitas	4	

1. Sauté onion and garlic until onion is soft.
2. Using a blender, puree all ingredients. Serve with pita bread or as a vegetable dip. Yield: 2 cups.

Lentil Burgers

dry lentils	¾ cup	180 mL	eggs, slightly beaten	2	
water	1½ cups	360 mL	oregano	¼ tsp	1.25 mL
finely chopped onion	⅓ cup	80 mL	oil	2 tbsp	30 mL
grated carrots	½ cup	120 mL	processed cheese (optional)	2 slices	
dry breadcrumbs	1½ cups	360 mL			

1. Add water to the lentils; bring to boil. Cover and simmer 15 minutes.
2. Add onion and carrots; cook about 15 minutes or until lentils are tender.
3. Cool slightly. Add crumbs, eggs, and oregano. Mix well.
4. Heat oil in large skillet. Drop lentil mixture, ½ cup (120 mL) at a time, into hot oil. Flatten to make patties.
5. Cook patties until firm, about 7 minutes on each side. If desired, top each patty with cheese and heat to melt cheese. (Four servings.)

Soybean–Corn–Tomato Casserole

cooked soybeans	2 cups	480 mL	garlic powder	¼ tsp	1.25 mL
whole kernel corn, drained	1 cup	240 mL	oregano	¼ tsp	1.25 mL
cooked tomatoes	1 cup	240 mL	basil leaves	½ tsp	2.5 mL
flour	1 tsp	5 mL	cheese, shredded	1 oz.	28 g

1. Set oven at 375°F (190°C).
2. Arrange beans and corn in alternate layers in a 1-quart (1-liter) greased baking dish.
3. Mash tomatoes with a fork; reserve 2 tbsp (30 mL) tomato juice.
4. Mix flour and seasonings in small saucepan. Combine reserved tomato juice and flour; add to tomatoes.
5. Heat, stirring until mixture boils.
6. Pour hot sauce over vegetables and bake about 20 minutes until heated through. During the last 5 minutes, sprinkle with cheese. Season. (Four servings.)

Stuffed Peppers

oil	1 tbsp	15 mL	cooked beans, mashed (e.g., kidney, pea, garbanzo)	1½ cups	360 mL
onion, chopped	¼ cup	60 mL	basil	½ tsp	2.5 mL
celery, chopped	¼ cup	60 mL	cheddar cheese, grated	⅓ cup	80 mL
cooked tomatoes	1 cup	240 mL	green peppers, seeded	3	

1. Set oven at 400°F (205°C).
2. Sauté onion and celery in oil until onion is lightly browned.
3. Add tomatoes, beans, and seasonings. Remove from heat and add cheese.
4. Fill the pepper halves with mixture.
5. Place peppers in an oblong baking pan with about 1 inch (2.54 mL) hot water in the bottom of the pan. Cover.
6. Bake 15 minutes; uncover and bake 10 to 15 minutes longer until peppers are just tender. Keep water in the pan. Season. (Three servings.)

Tamale Pie

Filling:

margarine	½ tbsp	7.5 mL	meat stock	¼ cup	60 mL
diced onion	¼ cup	60 mL	chili powder	¾ tsp	4 mL
cooked kidney beans	1 cup	240 mL	chopped olives (optional)	2 tbsp	30 mL
tomato soup	⅜ cup	90 mL	grated cheddar cheese	2 tbsp	30 mL

Cornbread Topping:

flour	2 tbsp	30 mL	buttermilk	¼ cup	60 mL
baking soda	1 tsp	0.63 mL	egg, beaten	½	
cornmeal	3 tbsp	45 mL	melted margarine	1 tbsp	15 mL

1. Set oven at 425°F (220°C).
2. Brown the onion in the fat. Add all ingredients except the cheese and simmer for about 5 minutes. Pour into two 6-oz. (180-mL) greased custard dishes. Sprinkle with cheese.
3. Sift the flour, baking soda, and salt together. Mix the cornmeal with the dry ingredients.
4. Combine the buttermilk, beaten egg, and melted fat and add to dry ingredients. Mix just enough to moisten. Spread batter over bean mixture.
5. Bake 20 minutes or until cornbread is golden brown. Season. (Two servings.)

APPETIZERS

Bean Salad

wax beans, cooked	⅓ cup	80 mL	vinegar	1 tbsp	15 mL
green beans, cooked	⅓ cup	80 mL	oil	2 tbsp	30 mL
kidney beans, cooked	1 cup	80 mL	sugar	½ tsp	2.5 mL
finely chopped onion	1 tbsp	15 mL	lettuce leaves	2–3	
finely chopped celery	2 tbsp	30 mL			

1. Mix beans and vegetables.
2. Beat vinegar, oil, and sugar. Add to vegetables, mixing gently.
3. Refrigerate for at least 1 hour. Spoon mixture onto lettuce leaves. Season. Chill. (Two to three servings.)

Black Bean Salsa

black beans, cooked	½ cup	120 mL	corn	½ cup	120 mL
tomato, chopped	1 cup	240 mL	cilantro, finely chopped	½ cup	120 mL
onion, finely chopped	¼ cup	60 mL	lemon juice	1 tbsp	15 mL
bell pepper, finely chopped	½ cup	120 mL	oil	1 tbsp	15 mL

1. Rinse beans and chop all vegetables except corn.
2. Combine all ingredients in a bowl. Chill before serving. (Six servings.)

TOFU RECIPES[4]

Korean Tofu Appetizer[5]

1. Place 12 oz. (340 g) tofu block, extra firm, on serving dish.
2. Sprinkle tofu with one sliced green onion and 1 tablespoon (15 mlL) light soy sauce.
3. Slice to serve with crackers.

[4] Soybean curd (tofu) is coagulated soy protein. Wash and drain before adding to a recipe. Its most commonly available varieties are extra firm, firm, and soft, which have uses specific to individual recipes.
[5] Quick to fix.

Tofu Burgers

tofu	6 oz.	170 g	parmesan cheese, grated	2 tsp	10 mL
egg	1		pepper	¼ tsp	1.25 mL
breadcrumbs	½ cup	120 mL	oregano	¼ tsp	1.25 mL
onion, minced	2 tbsp	30 mL	cayenne	dash	
garlic, minced	1 tsp	5 mL	oil, vegetable	1 tbsp	15 mL

1. Combine all ingredients in a bowl and stir until well mixed.
2. Heat oil in 10- to 12-inch skillet.
3. Form the tofu mixture into 4 patties and fry to brown both sides.
4. Place on baking sheet in 350°F (175°C) oven for 10 to 15 minutes. If desired, serve with lettuce and tomato in a bun. (Four servings.)

Stir-Fried Tofu with Spinach

raw rice	1 cup	240 mL	chopped spinach	5 oz.	142 g
tofu	½ lb.	227 g	low-sodium soy sauce	½–1 tbsp	7–15 mL
peanut oil	2 tsp	10 mL			

1. Cook rice. Maintain temperature at or above 140°F (60°C).
2. In a large skillet, sauté tofu cubes in oil about 5 minutes. Stir gently. Push cubes to center and spread spinach around edge.
3. Sprinkle with soy sauce and cover. Steam mixture until spinach has just wilted.
4. Season. Serve mixture over hot rice. (Two servings.)

Pineapple Banana Shake

soft tofu	4–6 oz.	114–170 g	orange juice	½ cup	120 mL
crushed pineapple	1 cup	240 mL	banana	½	

Place all ingredients in a blender and process until smooth. If too thick, add more fruit juice. Keep refrigerated. Serve chilled. Yield: 2 cups (480 mL).

SUMMARY QUESTIONS—PLANT PROTEINS

1. In cooking dried beans:
   a. What steps are important in obtaining a tender product?

   b. What common ingredients, if added too early in the cooking process, will cause the beans to harden?

   c. In cooking beans, how are the pectin, protein, and starch of the beans changed?

2. Identify generalizations that may be made concerning the use of a crock pot for cooking beans or peas.

3. Regarding the use of dried beans:
   a. One cup of dried beans is equal to how many cups of cooked beans?

   b. Contrast the cost of dried beans to that of canned beans. When might canned products be advantageous?

4. One cup of cooked, dried beans has approximately how many grams of protein? What other major nutrients do legumes contribute? What is the possible allergen component?

5. List commonly used food combinations that illustrate the principle of mutual supplementation.

6. Complete the following chart:

Food Product	Amino Acids[a]	
	High	Low
Grains		
Legumes		
Soybeans		
Nuts		
Seeds		
Lentils		

[a] Consult Appendix O.

7. Explore several cookbooks of other regions in the United States as well as other countries.
   a. Attach a list of vegetable protein dishes and characteristic meals from each region/country.

   b. Discuss how principles of mutual supplementation of proteins have been applied in these dishes and meals.

c. Evaluate the potential protein quality of these cookbook vegetable protein dishes.

8. Discuss other nutritional dimensions (e.g., saturated fat, cholesterol, minerals, vitamins) that should be considered when substituting plant protein for animal protein in the diet.

9. Why are legumes considered the foundation of a strict vegetarian diet?

10. If an individual has an allergy to legumes, what foods cannot be consumed?

11. Discuss economic benefits of a plant-based diet.

12. Discuss culinary variation offered by utilizing a plant-based cuisine.

13. A friend is switching to a lacto-ovo-vegetarian diet after 20 years on a "typical American diet." Summarize key points you would suggest about the nutritional quality of the new diet. How would your advice differ if the friend were changing to a strict vegetarian regimen?

Dietitian's Note

See Appendices and websites.

F. Eggs and Egg Products

I do not like them, Sam-I-am. I do not like green eggs and ham.

— **Dr. Seuss**

Objectives

To identify characteristics indicative of egg quality and relate these to use of eggs in food preparation
To observe the time–temperature relationships that occur during the coagulation of egg proteins
To know and apply temperature standards for safe handling of cooked egg products
To describe the effect of manipulation, especially stirring and rate of heating on the coagulation temperature of egg mixtures
To describe the effect of ingredients and their proportions on the coagulation of egg mixtures
To demonstrate preparation of an egg white foam
To delineate factors that affect both foam volume and stability
To relate egg characteristics to uses of eggs in food preparation
To apply principles of the combination of starch and egg cookery in food preparation
To appraise the nutritive, sanitary, and economic dimensions of eggs and egg substitutes
To identify egg allergies and acceptable recipe alternatives

References

Appendices E, H-I, H-II, L-I, L-II, N
www.aeb.org — American Egg Board
www.usda.gov
http://www.ams.usda.gov/howtobuy/eggs.htm
http://www.fightbac.org/heatitup.cfm

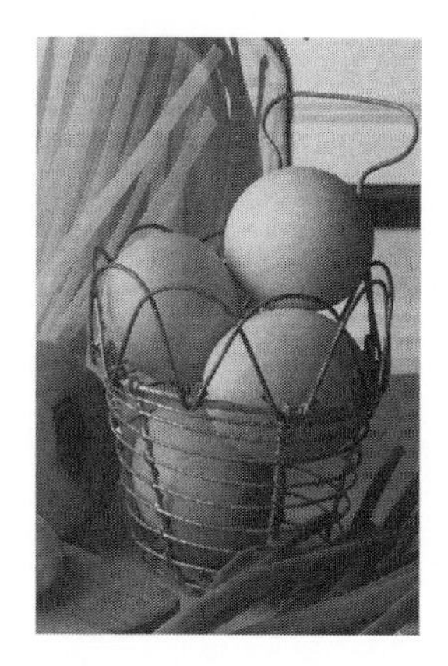

EGGS.
Courtesy: SYSCO® Incorporated.

Terms

Beat	Egg allergy	Interbonding	Soft peak
Cholesterol	Egg substitutes	Intrabonding	Stiff peak
Coagulation	Foam, foamy	Poach	Syneresis
Curdling	Fold	*Salmonella*	Weeping
Dry peak	Fry	Sol/Gel	Whip

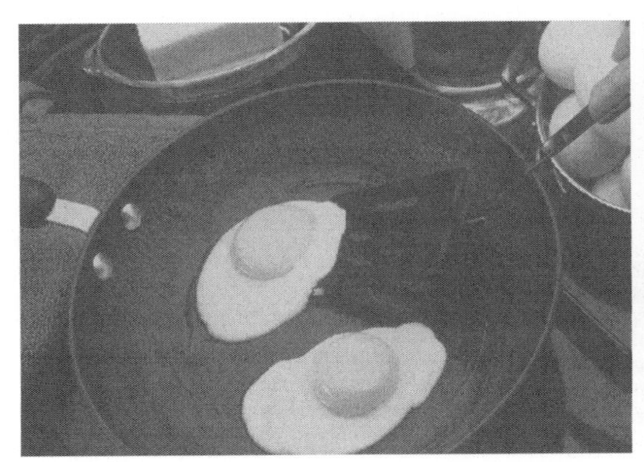

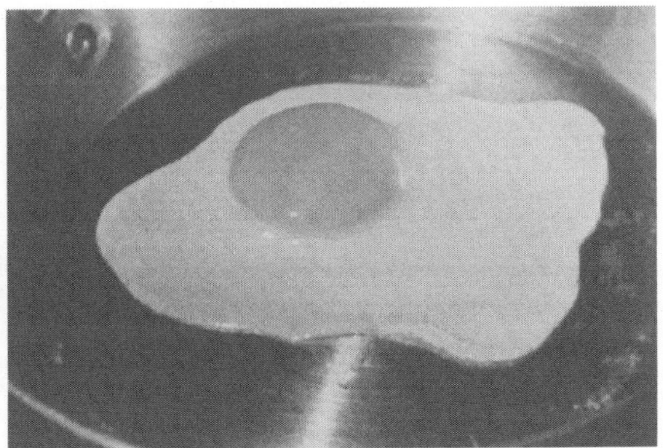

Fresh Eggs with Upstanding Yolks and Firm Whites (*Courtesy*: American Egg Board) Contrasted (Right) to Older Egg (Courtesy: USDA).

Ensuring the Safety of Eggs

- Keep eggs refrigerated until ready to use. Instead of being left at room temperature, eggs may be placed in warm water to warm up prior to beating.
- Check final temperature of cooked product.
- DO NOT taste any egg product until firm:
  whites 144–149°F (62–65°C);
  yolks 144–158°C (62–70°C).
  Cook to 160°F (71°C).

AMERICAN EGG BOARD

Egg Doneness Guidelines

Scrambled eggs, omelets, and frittatas		Cook until the eggs are thickened and no visible liquid egg remains.
Fried eggs		To cook both sides and increase the temperature the eggs reach, cook slowly, and either baste the eggs, cover the pan with a lid, or turn the eggs. Cook until the whites are completely set and the yolks begin to thicken but are not hard.
Soft-cooked eggs		Bring eggs and water to a full, rolling boil. Turn off the heat, cover the pan, and let the eggs sit in the hot water about 4 to 5 minutes.
Poached eggs		Cook in gently simmering water until the whites are completely set and the yolks begin to thicken but are not hard, about 3 to 5 minutes. Avoid precooking and reheating poached eggs.
Soft (stirred) custards, including cream pie, eggnog, and ice cream bases		Cook until thick enough to coat a metal spoon with a thin film and a thermometer shows 160°F or higher. After cooking, cool quickly by setting the pan in ice or cold water and stirring for a few minutes. Cover and refrigerate to chill thoroughly, at least 1 hour.

EXERCISE 1: EGG QUALITY

Procedure

1. Place eggs of various freshness (age) in a bowl of water.
2. Note which eggs float, and which sink.
3. Carefully open each egg and place each in a saucer. Observe characteristics of the white and yolk.
4. Record observations and summarize conclusions.

Whole Egg in Water	Description of White	Description of Yolk

Conclusions:

1. Why did some eggs float? Explain.

2. What other methods are used for judging the quality of eggs?

EXERCISE 2: COAGULATION OF EGG PROTEIN IN BAKED AND STIRRED CUSTARD

BASIC EGG CUSTARD—FOR BAKED AND STIRRED CUSTARD

milk	3 cups	720 mL	sugar	⅓ cup	80 mL
eggs, large	3		vanilla	1 tsp	5 mL

PROCEDURE FOR BOTH BAKED AND STIRRED CUSTARDS

1. Calibrate thermometer and set oven at 400°F (205°C). Label small paper cups for stirred custard samples.
2. Scald milk in top of double boiler over hot water.
3. Place egg and sugar into a medium-sized mixing bowl and mix slightly. Pour scalded milk slowly into the mixture, stirring constantly. Add vanilla.

Use the mixture for BOTH the *Baked* and *Stirred Custard* preparations as directed.

BAKED CUSTARD[1]

1. Fill two custard cups three-quarters full of the *Basic Egg Custard* recipe. Reserve the remainder of the mixture for the *Stirred Custard*.
2. Place one cup in a pan of hot water, with water level even with the custard.
3. Place the second cup in a pan or on a cookie sheet with no water.
4. Bake for 25 minutes, or until the sample cooked in water is fully cooked. (Fully cooked is determined by inserting a metal knife into the custard, halfway between the edge and center. When the knife comes out clean, the custard is done.)
5. Label and cool the baked samples. Record observations of appearance, texture, and consistency, using palatability terms provided.

[1] Refer to chapter on Microwave Cooking for microwave recipes.

Baked Custard

	Appearance	Texture	Consistency
Baked in water bath			
Baked without water			
Baked in microwave			

Conclusions:

PALATABILITY TERMS

APPEARANCE	TEXTURE	CONSISTENCY
Glossy	Smooth	Thin
Dull	Velvety	Watery
Shiny	Lumpy	Slightly thickened
	Curdled	Thick
	Porous	Gel-like
		Firm

STIRRED CUSTARD

For **class use**, follow steps 1 to 8.

1. Pour the remainder of the *Basic Egg Custard* recipe mixture (remainder from *Baked Egg Custard*) back into the top of the double boiler.
2. Place cold water in the bottom of the double boiler at a level that does not touch the top pan.
3. Begin to cook the mixture, stirring as soon as it is placed over the heat.
4. After the water on the bottom starts to boil, turn the heat to medium-low to maintain a simmer. Do not boil.
5. Hold the calibrated thermometer in the center of the mixture, resting it on the bottom of the top pan. Do not remove the thermometer while the mixture is cooking.
6. Stir the mixture continuously, while quickly removing samples (placing samples in paper cups) with a metal spoon at designated temperatures.
7. While removing samples, note at what temperature the metal spoon is slightly coated and at what temperature the coating becomes heavy and velvety. Record observations at each temperature.
8. After the custard has reached maximum thickness, continue to cook it until it curdles. Record the curdling temperature.

(For **culinary use**, follow steps 1 to 4. Then cook for about 20 minutes until mix coats spoon. Chill quickly by placing pan in a bowl of ice water. Transfer to serving bowl, cover with plastic wrap, and place in refrigerator 2 to 3 hours.)

9. Label and cool all samples. Record observations and summarize the effect of increasing temperature on egg protein, appearance, texture, and consistency, using appropriate palatability terms.

Sample Temperature	Appearance	Texture	Consistency
177°F (81°C)			
181.4°F (83°C)			
183°F (84°C)			
185°F (85°C)			
187°F (86°C)			
188.6°F (87°C)			
190.4°F (88°C)			
Curdled			

Conclusions:

1. Protein is the component responsible for the functional properties of eggs in food preparation.
   a. Describe how protein is dispersed in a raw egg (a sol/a gel).

   b. Describe how protein is dispersed in a cooked egg (a sol/a gel).

   c. Explain how heat, including high heat, affects egg protein.

   d. At what temperature do egg yolks and egg whites coagulate?

2. What changes in egg protein structure take place while the egg mixture is cooking:
   a. If prepared as a stirred custard?

   b. If prepared as a baked custard?

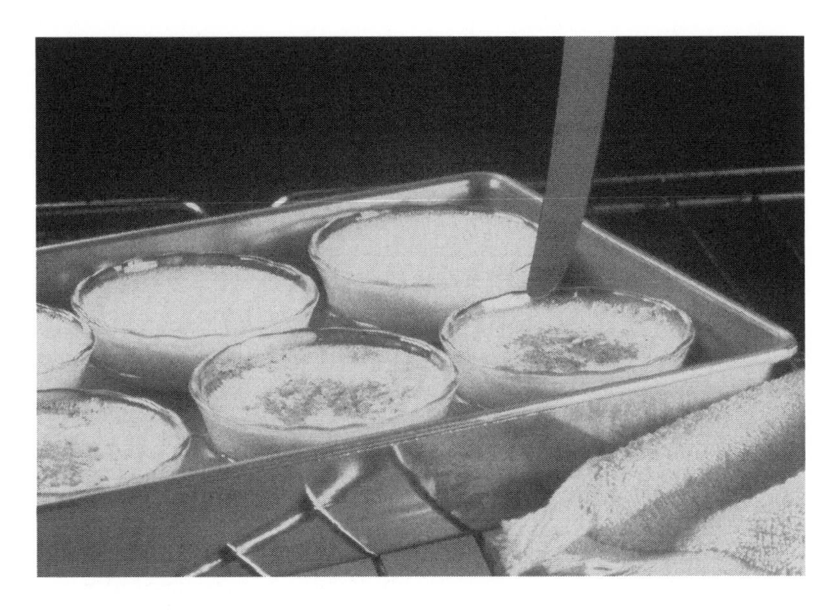

Testing Egg Custard.
Courtesy: American Egg Board.

3. Describe what occurs in terms of structure, when the temperature of the custard is raised above the coagulation point of the egg protein.

4. How does the speed of cooking a stirred custard affect coagulation temperature? Explain any adverse affect speed of cooking has on the product.

5. Does a fully cooked baked custard become appreciably thicker upon cooling? Explain.

6. What is the purpose of using a water bath when baking custard? For what other products would a water bath be beneficial?

EXERCISE 3: EGG WHITE FOAMS

PROCEDURE

1. Separate two eggs, placing whites and yolks into separate bowls.
2. Beat egg whites with rotary or electric beater to designated stage of foam. Record observations on foam development as beating continues.
3. Beat yolks until thick and lemon colored, then fold yolks into beaten whites.
4. Summarize observations; contrast effect of beating egg whites and yolks.

Stage of Foam	Volume	Description	Comments
Coarse foam			
Foamy			
Soft peak			
Stiff peak			
Dry foam			

Conclusions:

1. Describe the structural formation of the protein in an egg white foam.

2. What properties or characteristics of egg whites make them useful as leavening agents?

3. Is a foam beaten to the dry stage as effective a leavening agent as a stiff-peak foam? Explain.

4. Describe the process of folding beaten yolks into beaten whites.

5. Contrast volume obtained by beating egg yolks until thick to that of egg white beaten to stiff peaks.

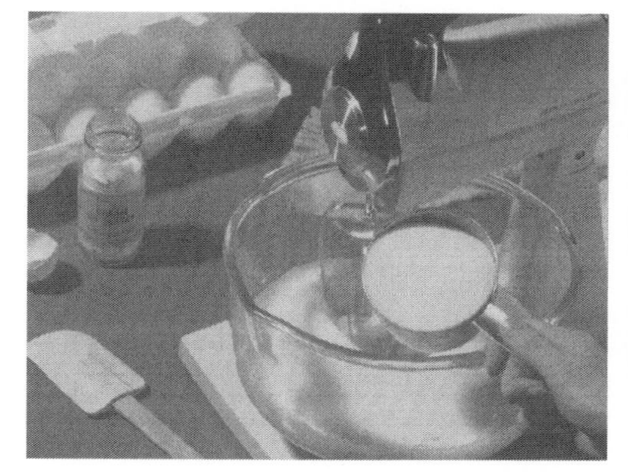

Courtesy: American Egg Board.

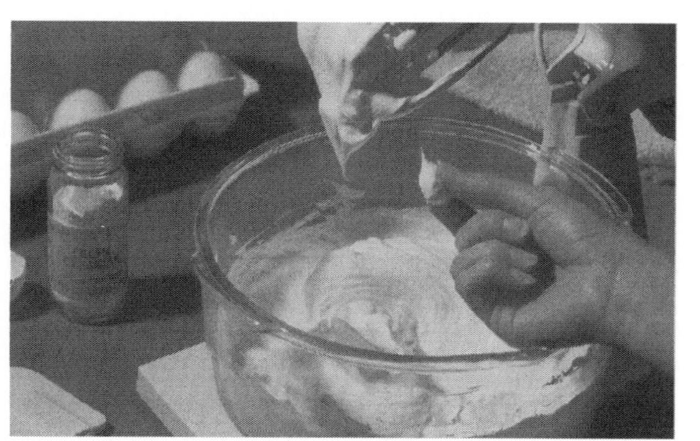

Courtesy: American Egg Board.

Egg Component	Volume	Explanation
Beaten yolks		
Whites beaten to stiff peaks		

EXERCISE 4: EFFECT OF ADDED SUBSTANCES ON EGG WHITE FOAM[2]

PROCEDURE

1. Measure the volume of one egg white; place it in a 1-quart (or liter) bowl.
2. Add one of the assigned ingredients to each white, as directed.
3. Beat each mixture for 2 minutes, or until the foam reaches a stiff-peak stage.
4. Carefully measure the final volume and display the foam.
5. Record observations on foam volume, stability, and general appearance.
6. Hold samples for 10 minutes and re-evaluate the foam characteristics.

Ingredient—1 Egg White Plus:	Initial Volume	Final Volume	Observations—Stability, Appearance	Re-evaluation after 10 Minutes
¼ tsp (1.25 mL) cream of tartar, added initially				
¼ tsp (1.25 mL) cream of tartar, added at foamy stage				
2 tbsp (30 mL) sugar, added initially				
2 tbsp (30 mL) sugar, added at soft-peak stage				
1 tbsp (15 mL) water, added initially				
⅛ tsp (0.63 mL) oil, added initially				

Conclusions:

[2] While eggs at room temperature beat more easily and to a greater volume, microbiological considerations caution that eggs should not be left at room temperature. Instead, allow eggs to warm up by placing them in a bowl of warm water for several minutes prior to preparing an egg white foam.

EXERCISE 5: EFFECT OF COOKING INTENSITY ON EGG PROTEIN

PROCEDURE

Cook refrigerated egg(s) according to assigned procedure listed below, using assigned cooking intensity (time and temperature) as directed. Check the final temperature of the product and record palatability evaluations.

METHODS OF COOKING EGGS[3]

Eggs Cooked in Shell (Soft or Hard Cooked): Place whole egg in small saucepan, with water to cover.
Eggs Cooked in Water (Poached): Fill shallow pan with water, twice the depth of egg. Bring water to specified temperature. Remove egg from shell and place in custard cup. Swirl water with a spoon and carefully drop egg into vortex.
Eggs Cooked in Fat (Fried): Place 1 tsp (5 mL) fat in a small frying pan, melt over low heat. Remove egg from shell and place in pan.
Egg Mixture (Scrambled): Mix 2 eggs and 2 tbsp (30 mL) milk. If scrambling in frying pan, add 1 tsp (5 mL) margarine and melt or use nonstick spray. Add egg mixture. If using double boiler, place egg mixture in top over simmering water in bottom pan. Gently stir mixture until it is firm and moist.
Baked Eggs (Shirred): Break egg into lightly greased custard cup. Season as desired and add ½ tsp (2.5 mL) margarine to egg. Bake uncovered at 350°F (175°C).

Evaluation[4] of Eggs Cooked in Various Ways

Procedure	Cooking Time (min.)	Final Temp.	White	Yolk	Texture/ Tenderness
Eggs cooked in shell Simmer	15				
Simmer	25				
Boil	15				
Boil	20				
Heat to boiling. Turn off heat. Let stand.	15				
Heat to boiling. Turn off heat. Let stand.	25				

[3] Refer to chapter on Microwave Cooking for microwave recipes.
[4] Do not taste eggs that have not reached 145°F (63°C). For undercooked eggs, observe texture.

Procedure	Cooking Time (min.)	Final Temp.	White	Yolk	Texture/ Tenderness
Eggs cooked in water—poached Simmer	7				
Simmer: water + 1 tsp (5 mL) vinegar	7				
Boil	7				
Eggs cooked in fat (fried) LOW-MED heat, uncovered	5				
HIGH heat, uncovered	4				
LOW heat, covered + 1 tbsp (15 mL) water	5				
Egg mixtures (scramble) Frying pan: LOW heat	3–5				
Frying pan: HIGH heat	4				
Double boiler: until firm	6–8				
Baked eggs (shirred) Bake	10–15				
Bake	25				

EXERCISE 6: CHARACTERISTICS OF COOKED MODIFIED EGG MIXTURES[5]

PROCEDURE

1. Using standard procedures, pan-fry or scramble 2 whole eggs, 3 whites, or ½ cup (120 mL) commercial cholesterol-free egg product.
2. Record observations of texture, flavor, appearance, and nutritive values.

[5] Observe temperature precautions for tasting cooked eggs, although cholesterol-free egg mix is pasteurized.

Egg/Egg Product	Appearance	Texture	Flavor	Cholesterol	Fat (g)	Protein (g)
Pan-fried egg						
Whole eggs						
Egg whites						
Cholesterol-free						
Scrambled						
Whole + 1 tbsp (15 mL) milk						
Whites + 1 yolk + 1 tbsp (15 mL) milk						
Cholesterol-free						

EXERCISE 7: COMBINING STARCH AND EGGS AS THICKENERS IN ONE PRODUCT—SOUFFLÉ

PROCEDURE

1. Prepare a soufflé that uses both starch and egg protein for thickening and structure, and egg white for leavening.
2. Evaluate the palatability of soufflé based on the following criteria.
3. Analyze the starch and protein component of the product structure (sol, gel).

	Palatability
Texture	
Consistency	
Volume	
Flavor	

Component	Uncooked Product	Hot, Cooked Product
Starch		
Protein, egg white		
Protein, egg yolk		

1. Explain how the principles of starch gelatinization were applied in preparing the starch/egg product.

2. Explain how the principles of egg protein coagulation were applied.

Soufflé Recipes[6]

Cheese Soufflé

margarine	2 tbsp	30 mL	cheddar cheese, grated	½ cup	120 mL
flour	1½ tbsp	22.5 mL	eggs, separated	2	
milk	½ cup	120 mL			

1. Set oven at 325°F (163°C).
2. Prepare a thickened sauce with flour and milk.
3. Add the cheese and stir the mixture over low heat until the cheese melts.
4. In a small bowl, beat egg yolk slightly with a fork.
5. Slowly add a little of the hot mixture to yolks, stirring to blend. Then add the warmed egg mixture to the cheese sauce. Mix thoroughly. Set aside to cool slightly.
6. Beat the egg whites until stiff.
7. Gradually fold the cheese–yolk mixture into the beaten whites.
8. Pour the mixture into two 10-oz. (300-mL) ungreased baking dishes. To make a "high hat" on a soufflé, use a knife point and trace a circular groove on the top of mixture, about 1 inch (2.54 cm) from the edge.
9. Bake 20 minutes or until a knife inserted in the center comes out clean. If a water bath is used, set oven at 375°F (190°C). (Two servings.)

[6] Recipes may contain known allergens. See Appendix E.

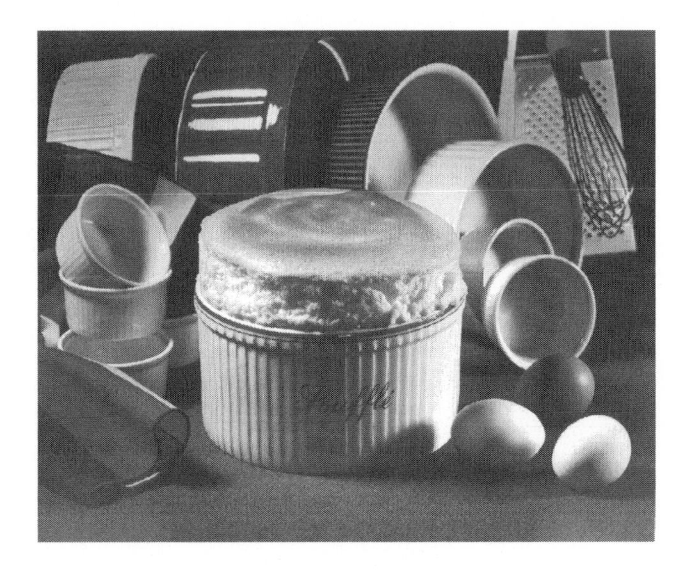

CHEESE SOUFFLÉ.
Courtesy: American Egg Board.

Chili Rellenos

green chilies, seeded, deveined, and chopped	4 oz.	114 g	eggs, separated	2	
jack cheese, grated	⅓ lb.	151 g	evaporated milk	½ cup	120 mL
			flour	2 tbsp	30 mL

1. Set oven at 325°F (165°C).
2. Place a layer of chilies in three 10-oz. (300-mL) greased baking dishes.
3. Cover with a layer of cheese. Repeat.
4. Beat egg whites until stiff.
5. Beat evaporated milk, flour, and egg yolks until well blended.
6. Gently fold egg whites into yolk mixture (mixture will be thin).
7. Pour egg–milk mixture over chilies.
8. Bake 25 to 30 minutes or until custard has set. (Three servings.)

Chocolate Soufflé

flour	½ tbsp	7.5 mL	margarine (optional)	1 tsp	5 mL
sugar	3 tbsp	45 mL	vanilla	1 tsp	5 mL
milk	½ cup	120 mL	eggs, separated	2	
baking chocolate, grated	½ oz.	14 g			

1. Set oven at 325°F (165°C).
2. Mix flour and sugar in saucepan. Add milk and chocolate, stirring.
3. Heat, stirring constantly until thickened. Stir in margarine and vanilla. Set aside.
4. Beat yolks until thick and lemon colored. Slowly add the thickened milk to yolks, stirring constantly.
5. Beat egg whites until stiff.
6. Fold chocolate mixture into whites. Pour into three 6-oz. (180-mL) ungreased baking dishes or custard cups.
7. Bake 25 to 30 minutes, or until custard has set. (Three servings.)

Spoon Bread

milk	1½ cups	360 mL	sugar	1 tbsp	15 mL
cornmeal, white	⅓ cup	80 mL	baking powder	½ tsp	2.5 mL
margarine	1 tbsp	15 mL	eggs, separated	2	

1. Set oven at 325°F (165°C).
2. Scald milk in top of double boiler.
3. Stir in cornmeal gradually and cook over boiling water until thickened, stirring occasionally. If very thick, add ¼ cup (60 mL) milk.
4. Add fat, sugar, and baking powder; mix well.
5. Beat egg yolks until thick and lemon colored. Add hot cornmeal mixture slowly to beaten egg yolks, stirring to blend.
6. Beat egg whites until stiff.
7. Gently fold cornmeal mixture into beaten whites.
8. Spoon into six 4-oz. (120-mL) ungreased baking dishes.
9. Bake 30 minutes, or until custard has set. (Six servings.)

Tuna Soufflé

margarine	1 tbsp	15 mL	tuna, drained and flaked[a]	3 oz.	85 g
onion, minced	1 tsp	5 mL	paprika	dash	
flour	1½ tbsp	22.5 mL	eggs, separated	2	
milk	½ cup	120 mL			

[a] Canned salmon, chopped cooked shrimp, chicken, or ham may be used.

1. Set oven at 325°F (165°C).
2. Melt fat and sauté onion. Blend in flour.
3. Add milk gradually and cook, stirring constantly until mixture thickens. Remove from heat and stir in tuna and paprika.
4. Beat egg yolks until thick and lemon colored. Slowly add hot tuna mixture to yolks, stirring constantly.
5. Beat egg whites until stiff.
6. Gently fold tuna–yolk mixture into beaten whites. Spoon into two 10-oz. (300-mL) or four 4-oz. (120-mL) ungreased baking dishes.
7. Bake 30 minutes, or until custard has set. (Three servings.)

Vegetable Soufflé[7]

margarine	2 tbsp	30 mL	cooked vegetable, chopped	1 cup	240 mL
milk	¾ cup	180 mL	eggs, separated	2	
flour	2 tbsp	30 mL			

1. Set oven at 325°F (165°C).
2. Melt fat. Stir in flour. Gradually stir in milk and cook, stirring constantly, until thickened. Add vegetable; remove from heat.
3. In a small bowl, beat egg yolks slightly.
4. Slowly add some of the vegetable mixture to yolks. Slowly pour warmed yolk mixture back into vegetable mixture, stirring constantly. Set aside to cool slightly.
5. In larger bowl, beat egg whites just until stiff. Gently fold vegetable–yolk mixture into egg whites; spoon into four 4-oz. (120-mL) ungreased baking dishes.
6. Bake 25 to 30 minutes, or until puffy, golden brown, and custard has set. (Three to four servings.)

EXERCISE 8: OTHER EGG RECIPES

PROCEDURE

1. Prepare egg dishes as assigned below.
2. Evaluate the palatability of each dish based on the following criteria.

	Palatability		
Characteristics	Stuffed Eggs	Eggs Benedict	Other as Assigned
Appearance			
Texture			
Flavor			

Stuffed Eggs

hard cooked eggs	3	30 mL	dry mustard	dash	2.5 mL
mayonnaise	2 tbsp		pepper	dash	
salt	dash		onion, minced	½ tsp	

1. Cut the cooked eggs in half lengthwise. Remove yolks.
2. Mash yolks with remaining ingredients.
3. Refill whites and top with a sprinkle of paprika.

[7] The addition of ¼ c (60 ml) grated cheddar cheese enhances flavor.

Eggs Benedict

eggs	8	Canadian bacon	8 slices
English muffin	4		

1. Heat water over high heat until it boils, then turn heat to medium-low.
2. Break each egg separately into a cup and slip it into a simmering 1 inch (2.54 mL) of water. Repeat for all eight eggs.
3. Cover skillet and cook approximately 5 minutes until white and yolk are thick.
4. While eggs are cooking, broil muffin halves topped with Canadian bacon.
5. Place 1 egg on each muffin. Top with hollandaise sauce.

Cooked Hollandaise Sauce

egg yolks	3		butter, cold, cut in 16 pieces	½ cup	120 mL
water	¼ cup	60 mL	paprika	dash	
lemon juice	2 tbsp	30 mL	red pepper	dash	

1. In a small saucepan, beat together egg yolks, water, and lemon juice.
2. Cook over **very** low heat, stirring constantly, until yolk mixture bubbles at edges.
3. Stir in butter, 1 piece at a time, until melted and sauce is thickened.
4. Stir in seasonings. Remove from heat. Cover and chill if not using immediately. Yield: ¾ cup (180 mL). (Adapted from American Egg Board.)

SUMMARY QUESTIONS—EGGS AND EGG PRODUCTS

1. Relating to egg quality:
   a. List three uses for which older eggs are satisfactory.

   b. List three products for which high egg quality is essential.

2. What causes the egg white to become thinner with age? Does this thinning affect the thickening power of eggs? The foaming power of eggs? Explain.

3. How does an increase in the following ingredients of a soft custard affect the coagulation temperature? Soft custard basic recipe: 2 cups (480 mL) milk, 2 large eggs, ¼ cup (60 mL) sugar.

Added Ingredient	Change in Coagulation Temperature	Explanation
+ 2 tbsp (30 mL) sugar		
+ ⅓ cup (80 mL) milk		
+ 1 egg		

4. Outline briefly the major steps in the procedure for preparing a product that uses both starch and eggs as thickening agents.

5. Explain the technique used whereby eggs are successfully incorporated into a hot-starch mixture.

6. What sanitary problems might occur in the following situations:
   a. Use of cracked egg for eggnog.

   b. Storing dry powdered egg.

   c. Reconstituted powdered egg left unrefrigerated.

   d. Unpasteurized frozen eggs—whole, yolk, or white.

   e. Use of raw egg in Caesar salad dressing.

   f. Combining beaten egg white with fruit purée for a low-calorie dessert.

7. Investigate the current price of eggs per dozen. Which size is the "best buy"?

Size	Weight per Dozen	Cost per Dozen	Cost per Egg	Cost per Ounce
Extra large	27 oz. (765 g)			
Large	24 oz. (680 g)			
Medium	21 oz. (595 g)			

Conclusions:

8. Regarding egg substitutes used in the laboratory:
   a. Are they all cholesterol free? Explain.

   b. What is the composition and what additives are used in the cholesterol-free egg product?

   c. Identify how egg substitutes might be used in various food products.

   d. Compare the cost and nutritive value of these products relative to fresh eggs.

9. Predict the effect of using egg substitutes in place of egg whites for meringues.

10. Are egg substitutes acceptable for persons with egg allergies? Explain.

11. Record the nutritive value of one serving of the following foods, using recipes where provided. Circle those foods that contribute more than 10% RDA of a nutrient.

	Energy (kcal)	Protein (g)	Calcium (mg)	Iron (mg)	Vitamin A IU/RE	Thiamin (mg)	Riboflavin (mg)
Egg, 1 medium							
Baked custard							
Soufflé, cheese							
Pudding, vanilla							
RDA, 20-year-old male							
RDA, 20-year-old female							

Dietitian's Note

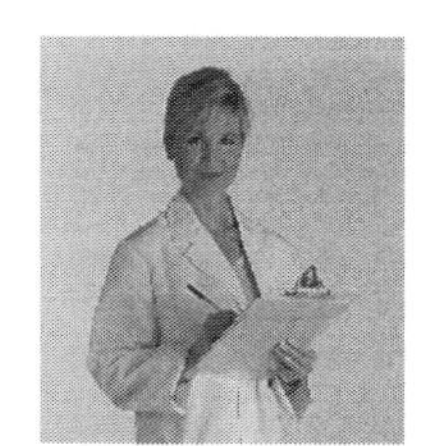

Recommendations are to limit eggs to four per week.
Only the yolks contain cholesterol.
www.aeb.org

G. Milk and Milk Products

I don't want the cheese, I just want to get out of the trap.

— **Spanish proverb**

Objectives

To recognize the variety of foods made from milk, and nondairy sources.
To appraise milk-product variations such as low-fat, fat-free, low-sodium cheeses and cheese products
To observe and describe reasons for coagulation of milk protein by several methods
To relate methods of coagulation to preparation and characteristics of several milk products
To observe, describe, and relate the effect of heat on natural and processed cheese
To appraise nutritive, palatability, sanitary, and economic characteristics of milk products
To identify lactose intolerance, milk protein allergies, and acceptable recipe alternatives

References

Appendix E, H-I
http://www.nationaldairycouncil.com
http://www.ampi.com

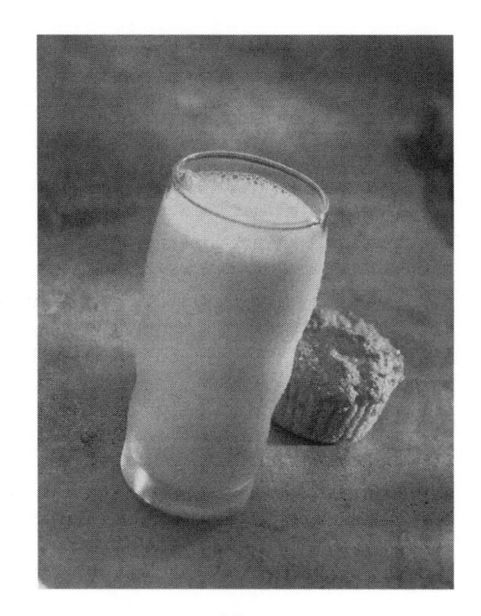

Milk.
Courtesy: SYSCO® Incorporated.

Terms

Campylobacteriosis
Casein
Cheese spread
Clot
Coagulation
Cold-pack cheese
Curd/Curdled
Enzyme/substrate
Homogenization
Imitation cheese
Kefir
Lactose intolerance
Listeriosis
Low-fat cheese
Low-sodium cheese
Milk allergy
Natural cheese
Pasteurization
Processed cheese
Rice milk/soy milk
Whey

EXERCISE 1: COMPARISON OF MILK AND NONDAIRY PRODUCTS

Procedure

1. Sample various milk or nondairy products, for example, low-fat, low-salt, nonfat, nonfat dry milk (NFDM), lactose-reduced, rice milk, soy milk, kefir, yogurt, and various aerosol "whipped-cream" products, as available.
2. Evaluate the palatability characteristic of each product (e.g., taste, consistency, acceptability).
3. Record the cost per serving and major nutrients supplied.
4. Summarize conclusions about the characteristics of the products, noting which may be considered the "best buy."

Sample Product	Palatability (your own ideas)	Cost/Serving	Major Nutrients

Conclusions:

1. Delineate the percent composition of whole milk:

Water: Carbohydrate: Fat: Protein: Minerals:

2. How does the percent of fat in whole milk compare with that of various other fluid milks?

3. Which of the sampled products contain no dairy products?

EXERCISE 2: COAGULATION OF MILK PROTEIN

A. ADDITION OF ACID

PROCEDURE

1. Bring 1 pint (480 mL) of whole milk to a boil.
2. Add 1 tbsp (15 mL) lemon juice to the hot milk.
3. Bring the milk to a boil again.
4. Strain the mixture through a double thickness of cheesecloth.
5. Carefully squeeze out excess water. Refrigerate the cheese. Yield: ½ cup (120 mL).

Questions:

1. Describe the appearance of the milk–acid mixture after it is boiled.

2. What is the composition of the soft precipitate (soft cheese) and the whey?

B. ACID PRODUCED BY BACTERIA (YOGURT)

PROCEDURE

1. Heat 1 quart (or liter) of milk to boiling. Pour into glass container.
2. Allow milk to cool to 111°F (44°C).
3. Stir 2 tbsp (30 mL) plain commercial yogurt into the milk.

4. Cover and leave the mixture undisturbed in a warm location 111°F (44°C), for 3 to 5 hours until set.
5. Refrigerate. Yield: 1 qt. (950 mL).

QUESTIONS:

1. Describe the final product. How does it differ from the product made by addition of acid in Part A?

2. In making yogurt, why is milk cooled to 111°F (44°C) before the bacterial culture is added?

3. How do the bacteria cause the coagulation of casein?

C. ENZYME ACTION (RENNIN)

PROCEDURE

1. Warm 2 cups (480 mL) milk slowly to lukewarm 111°F (44°C); remove from heat immediately.
2. Empty 1 package of rennin pudding into milk, stirring until dissolved, not more than 1 minute.
3. Immediately pour mixture into custard cups and leave undisturbed for 10 minutes. Refrigerate. (Four servings)

QUESTIONS:

1. Describe the final product.

2. What is the source of the enzyme rennin?

3. Identify the specific factors that are necessary for the optimum functioning of rennin.

4. How does the nutritive value of the product of rennin coagulation differ from that obtained when acid is used to coagulate casein? Why?

5. What other food products are made by rennin coagulation?

EXERCISE 3: COMBINING ACID FOODS WITH MILK

PROCEDURE

1. Using Alkacid test paper, or a pH meter, test the pH of milk and tomato juice.
2. Combine milk and tomato juice in the following five ways:
   a. Add ½ cup (120 mL) cold tomato juice to ½ cup (120 mL) hot milk.
   b. Add ½ cup (120 mL) cold tomato juice to ½ cup (120 mL) hot thickened[1] milk.
   c. Add ½ cup (120 mlL) cold tomato juice mixed with ⅛ tsp (.63 mL) soda to ½ cup (120 mL) hot milk.
   d. Add ½ cup (120 mL) hot thickened tomato juice to ½ cup (120 mL) cold milk.
   e. Add ½ cup (120 mL) hot tomato juice to ½ cup (120 mL) hot thickened milk.
3. Record the pH and evaluate the appearance of each mixture when first mixed.
4. Remove a sample of each mixture when the simmering temperature is reached. Evaluate the appearance.
5. Partially cover and cook the mixture over low heat for 15 minutes longer. Evaluate the appearance.
6. Based on experiments, draw conclusions regarding the best method for combining an acid ingredient with milk.

	Initial pH of Mixture	Appearance		
pH milk: pH tomato:		Initial Mixture	At Simmering	After 15 Minutes
Cold tomato to hot milk				
Cold tomato to hot thickened milk				
Cold tomato plus soda to hot milk				
Hot thickened tomato to cold milk				
Hot tomato to hot milk				

Conclusions:

[1] Where thickened tomato or milk product is required, use 1 tbsp (15 mL) fat and 1 tbsp (15 mL) flour.

PALATABILITY TERMS—CHEESE (FOR EXERCISE 4)								
FLAVOR				TEXTURE—CONSISTENCY				
Sharp	Soft	Bland	Sour	Soft	Semisoft	Crumbly	Moist	Firm
Strong	Acid	Mild	Sweet	Creamy	Curd	Granular	Dry	Hard
Salty								

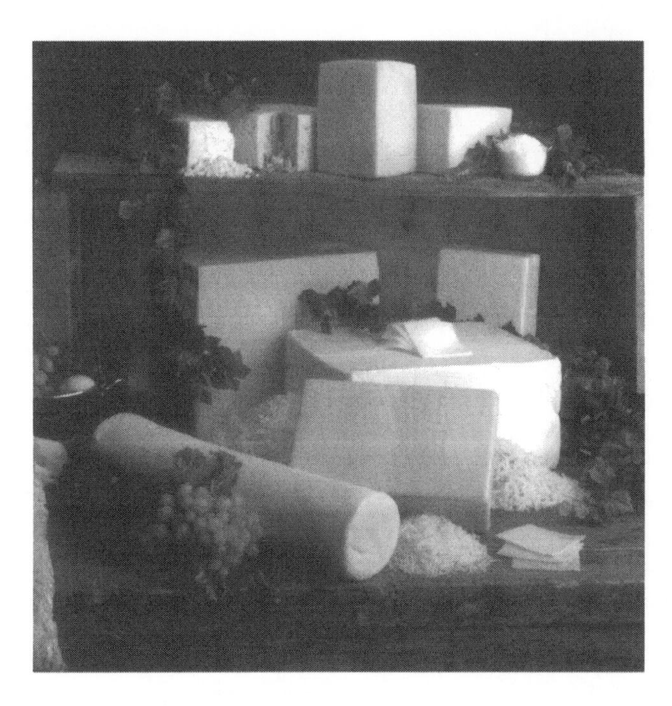

CHEESE.
Courtesy: SYSCO® Incorporated.

EXERCISE 4: COMPARISON OF CHEESE PRODUCTS

PROCEDURE

1. Sample cheese products on display, including cheeses as listed, or visit a grocery store to obtain use and cost data.
2. Complete the table, noting palatability characteristics, uses, and comparative cost.

Cheese Type	Name	Palatability	Uses	Cost/lb. (454 g)
Very hard	Parmesan			
	Other:			

(continued on next page)

Cheese Type	Name	Palatability	Uses	Cost/lb. (454 g)
Hard, ripened by bacteria	Cheddar			
	Edam–Gouda			
	Provolone			
	Other:			
Hard, ripened by bacteria (with eyes)	Swiss			
	Other:			
Semisoft, ripened by bacteria	Muenster			
	Monterey Jack			
	Other:			
Semisoft, ripened by blue mold (interior)	Roquefort			
	Blue			
	Other:			
Soft, ripened	Camembert			
	Other:			
Soft, unripened	Cottage			
	Cream			
	Neufchatel			
	Ricotta			
	Other:			
Cheese blends	Cold Pack			
	Other:			
Processed				
Low-salt				
Reduced-fat				

EXERCISE 5: EFFECT OF HEAT ON NATURAL AND PROCESSED CHEESE

PROCEDURE

1. Preheat oven to 350°F (175°C).
2. Place two slices of bread on a baking sheet.
3. On one slice, place 3 tbsp (45 mL) grated natural cheese; on the other slice, place 3 tbsp (45 mL) grated processed cheese. Cut each slice in half.
4. Place baking sheet on upper shelf of oven. Remove one-half slice of each sample as soon as the cheese melts (3 to 5 minutes). Describe the appearance and texture.
5. Bake the remaining halves for an additional 5 minutes. Describe the appearance and texture using the terms found below.

	Appearance	Texture
Natural cheese 5 minutes		
10 minutes		
Processed cheese 5 minutes		
10 minutes		

Conclusions:

PALATABILITY TERMS—COOKED CHEESE

APPEARANCE	TEXTURE–CONSISTENCY		
Homogeneous	Smooth	Tender	Stringy
Separated	Uniform	Tough	Elastic
Curdled			

1. How does the composition of processed and natural cheese differ?

2. Compare the effects of heat on the cooked samples of natural and processed cheese. Explain any differences.

3. What effect does extended cooking at high temperatures have on cheese?

SUMMARY QUESTIONS—MILK AND MILK PRODUCTS

1. In general, what are the most satisfactory methods of preventing coagulation of milk casein in recipes using vegetables?

2. Discuss the use of soda to prevent curdling of vegetable–milk combinations. Provide an example of when soda might be used.

3. In using a natural instead of processed cheese in a cheese sauce recipe, what special cooking techniques should be used to ensure a smooth sauce?

4. Did coagulation of casein play a role in the thickening of egg custards (egg and milk mixtures)? In the curdling of the overheated custard? Explain.

5. In the preparation of pizza, a hot oven temperature (450°F to 500°F, 230°C to 260°C) is used. How is the adverse effect of high heat on cheese protein minimized?

6. Based on laboratory experiments and readings, list the components in the following products that might cause coagulation of casein. How could coagulation be prevented?

Product	Factor Causing Coagulation	Prevention
Scalloped potatoes		
Cream of asparagus soup		
Ham slices baked in milk		
Milk–fruit juice beverage		

7. What practical suggestions can be offered to an individual who likes milk and milk products but needs to restrict calories?

8. Consult appropriate references and list several cheeses that are relatively low in calories and several that are low in sodium.

9. Complete the nutritive value chart.

Food	Energy (kcal)	Protein (g)	Fat (g)	Calcium (mg)	Vitamin A IU/RE	Riboflavin (mg)
Fluid milk (1 cup/240 mL)						
Whole milk						
2% milk						
½% milk						
Nonfat milk						
Sour cream (1 serving)						
Regular						
Low-fat						
Nonfat						
Yogurt (1 cup/240 mL)						
Regular						
Low-fat						
Nonfat						
Kefir						
Cottage cheese (1 cup/240 mL)						
Regular						
Low-fat						
Nonfat						

(continued on next page)

Food	Energy (kcal)	Protein (g)	Fat (g)	Calcium (mg)	Vitamin A IU/RE	Riboflavin (mg)
Cheddar cheese (1 oz./28 g)						
Reduced-fat						
Processed cheese						
Imitation cheese						

10. Account for differences in calcium content of cheddar cheese and cottage cheese.

11. What is lactose? How is lactose reduced in milks to provide more digestible milk?

12. In terms of sanitary quality, what problems may occur in the use of milk products? Explain.

13. Compare the cost of 10 g of protein from whole milk, cottage cheese, cheddar cheese, ground beef, and peanut butter.

14. What suggestions could be offered to someone on a low income about how to use nonfat dry milk? Consider especially the problem encountered by an individual who finds the taste unacceptable.

15. How does yogurt cheese differ from that made in Exercise 2A? Yogurt cheese is made as follows: 1 qt. (0.95 L) plain, low-fat yogurt is poured into a filter or cheesecloth-lined sieve, which is placed over a large bowl. Cover and refrigerate about 8 hours or overnight. The yield is 2 cups (480 mL) of a creamy spread or slightly less if a firmer cheese is desired. Season with herbs.

DIETITIAN'S NOTE

What is lactose intolerance?

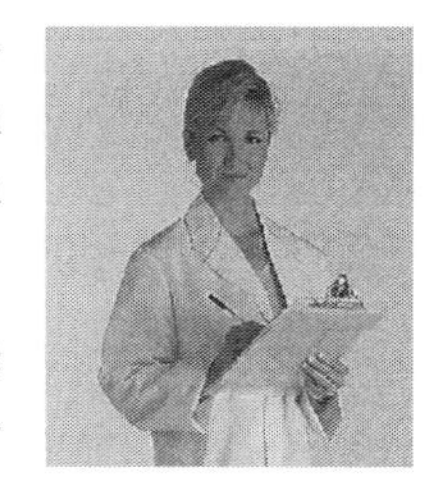

Lactose intolerance is the inability to digest significant amounts of lactose, the predominant sugar of milk. This inability results from a shortage of the enzyme lactase, which is normally produced by the cells that line the small intestine. Lactase breaks down milk sugar into simpler forms that can then be absorbed into the bloodstream.

When there is not enough lactase to digest the amount of lactose consumed, the results, although not usually dangerous, may be very distressing. While not all persons deficient in lactase have symptoms, those who do are considered to be lactose intolerant.

See: http://digestive.niddk.nih.gov/ddiseases/pubs/lactoseintolerance

What is the difference between lactose intolerance and milk allergy?

H. Fats and Oils

To lengthen thy life, lessen thy meals.

— Benjamin Franklin

Objectives

To illustrate some factors that affect the formation and stability of food emulsions
To apply the concepts of food emulsions to a variety of food products
To evaluate the effects of various fats and oils, and fat-replaced food products
To evaluate the palatability, cost, and nutritive value of fat-free and fat-reduced products
To identify fat and oil allergens and acceptable recipe alternatives

References

Appendices E, N
www.faseb.org
www.americanheart.org
www.eatright.org/Public/NutritionInformation/92_9292.cfm
www.iseo.org/foodfats.htm — Institute of Shortening and Edible Oils
www.ific.org

Terms

Calorie Restriction Diet
Cholesterol
Continuous phase
Cooked dressing
Dispersed phase
Emulsifier
Fat free
Fat substitute
French dressing
Lecithin
Mayonnaise
Nonstick cooking spray
Oil allergy
Pan fry
Polyunsaturated fat
Saturated fat
Sauté
Surface tension
Trans fat

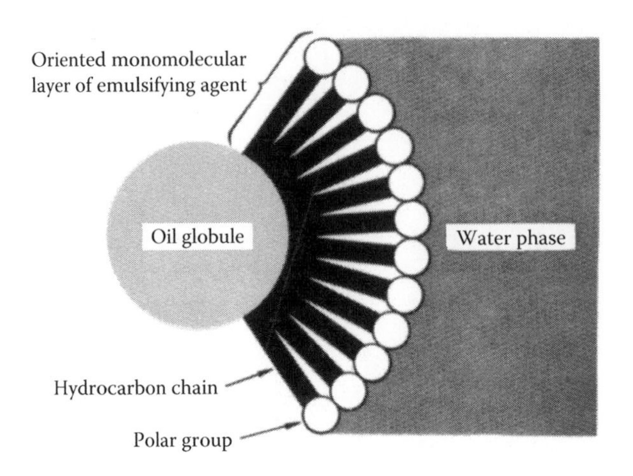

ORIENTATION OF EMULSIFYING AGENT IN AN OIL-IN-WATER EMULSION.

Source: Hartman, J.R. 1977. *Colloid Chemistry*. Boston: Houghton-Mifflin. Reprinted with permission.

EXERCISE 1: SEPARATION AND RATIO OF OIL AND ACID; EMULSIFIERS

PROCEDURE

1. Place vinegar and oil mixture in three test tubes as indicated.
2. Cover test tubes with plastic wrap and shake vigorously for 30 seconds.
3. Place test tubes in rack. Record the time that elapses before the mixtures separate.

Vinegar	Oil	Time of Separation
2 tsp (10 mL)	2 tsp (10 mL)	
1 tsp (5 mL)	2 tsp (10 mL)	
1 tsp (5 mL)	3 tsp (15 mL)	

4. Repeat experiment with standard (below) and emulsifiers.

Emulsifier	Time of Separation
Standard: 2 tsp (10 mL) oil and 1 tsp (5 mL) vinegar	
Standard + ⅛ tsp (0.63 mL) paprika	
Standard + ⅛ tsp (0.63 mL) dry mustard	
Standard + ⅛ tsp (0.63 mL) pepper	
Standard + beaten egg yolk	

Conclusion:

EXERCISE 2: APPLICATION OF PRINCIPLES TO SALAD DRESSINGS

PROCEDURE

1. Prepare assigned salad dressings and/or variations of recipes. (There may be other recipes to evaluate.)
2. Serve dressings on salad greens.
3. Evaluate products as to consistency and flavor and general acceptability.

Dressing	Consistency	Flavor	General Acceptability
French			
Mayonnaise			
Cooked dressing			

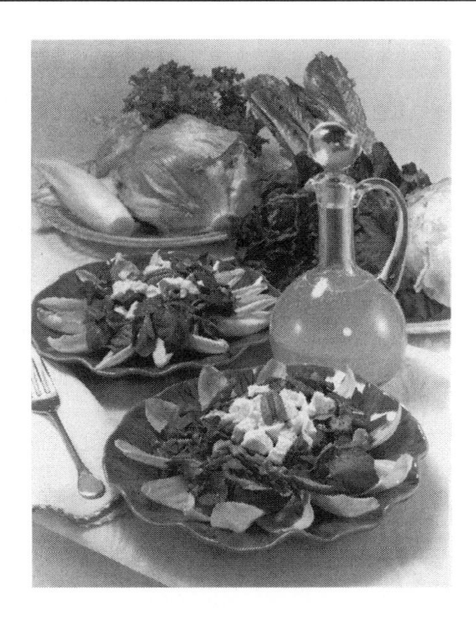

FRENCH DRESSING.
Courtesy: United Fresh Fruit and Vegetable Association.

SALAD DRESSING RECIPES

French Dressing

sugar	1 tsp	5 mL	vinegar	¼ cup	60 mL
paprika	¼ tsp	1.25 mL	salad oil	½ cup	120 ml
dry mustard	½ tsp	2.5 mL	clove garlic, crushed	1	
pepper	¼ tsp	1.25 mL			

1. Place all ingredients in a jar. Cover, shake well, and refrigerate. See variations.
2. Shake immediately prior to serving. Yield: ¾ cup (180 mL).

Salad dressing flavor variations

oil: safflower, canola, olive, sesame, hazelnut, walnut
acid: cider, white or wine vinegar; balsamic, rice, or fruit-flavored vinegars; citrus juice
herbs/spices: parsley, celery seed, tarragon, horseradish, curry, Worcestershire sauce, etc.
cheese: crumbed Roquefort, blue, parmesan

Cooked Mayonnaise[1,2]

egg yolks	2		dry mustard	1 tsp	5 mL
vinegar	2 tbsp	30 mL	pepper	dash	
water	2 tbsp	30 mL	salad oil	1 cup	240 mL
sugar	½ tsp	2.5 mL			

1. Place all ingredients except oil in a double boiler over simmering water. Stir constantly until mixture bubbles in one or two places.
2. Remove from heat and let stand 4 minutes.
3. Place cooked mixture in a blender and blend on high, or blend well with a whisk.
4. Very slowly, add oil and blend until mixture is thick and smooth.
5. Cover and refrigerate if not used immediately. Yield: 1¼ cups (300 mL).

Cooked Dressing

dry mustard	½ tsp	2.5 mL	milk	¾ cup	180 mL
sugar	1 tbsp	15 mL	egg, slightly beaten	1	
flour	2 tbsp	30 mL	vinegar or lemon juice	¼ cup	60 mL
paprika	⅛ tsp	0.63 mL	margarine	1 tbsp	15 mL

1. Mix dry ingredients, add milk and cook over direct heat, stirring until mixture boils.
2. Gradually add some of the hot starch to egg.
3. Add warmed egg–starch mixture to pan. Continue to cook over low heat until egg has thickened.
4. Gradually add vinegar and fat to mixture. Yield: 1 cup (240 mL).

[1] Recipes may contain known allergens. See Appendix E.
[2] Adapted from American Egg Board, Park Ridge, IL, 1991.

EXERCISE 3: FAT-FREE, FAT-REDUCED, AND FAT-REPLACED PRODUCTS

A. Calories, Cost, and Palatability of Foods with Various Fat Levels

Procedure

Evaluate and record the palatability characteristics, caloric value, and cost of the products assigned.

Product	Kcal/serving	Cost/serving	Palatability
Mayonnaise			
Salad dressing (mayo type) Fat-free			
Reduced-fat			
Salad dressing (non-mayo) Fat-free			
Reduced-fat			
Frozen dessert Fat-free			
Reduced-fat			
Baked product Fat-free			
Fat-replacement			
Cottage cheese Fat-free			
Reduced-fat			
Butter			
Butter blend			
Margarine Reduced-fat			
Fat-free			
Aerosol whipped cream			
Full-fat			
Fat-free			

1. Discuss nutritional advantages of using fat-free and fat-reduced products in the diet.

2. Discuss the various ways in which consumers could incorporate fat-free and/or fat-reduced foods in their diet if given the following situations:
   a. Consumers purchasing foods at the grocery

   b. Consumers choosing foods at restaurants

   c. Consumers preparing foods "from scratch" at home

3. Study the labels of commercial reduced- or fat-free dressings and compare with regular products. What additional ingredients and additives are used in the reduced- and/or no-fat products?

B. Fat-Replacement Ingredient Labeling

Procedure

1. Read labels on products containing fat replacements (may use labels from products in Part A and others).
2. Identify fat replacements by name (maltodextrin, Olean®, etc.).

Product	Fat Replacement

Suggest other reduced-fat products consumers might want to have available in the marketplace. Explain why replacements may not be possible in all the suggested products.

EXERCISE 4: COMPARISON OF DIETARY FATS

PROCEDURE

1. Complete chart, noting the percent saturated, polyunsaturated, and monounsaturated fat.
2. Record observations (e.g., composition, flavor) regarding those fats that were used in laboratory food preparation.

Comparison of Dietary Fats

Fat/Oil	% Saturated	% Polyunsaturated	% Monounsaturated	Observations
Canola oil				
Corn oil				
Olive oil				
Peanut oil				
Safflower oil				
Soybean oil				
Sunflower oil				
Butter				
Lard				
Margarine				
Vegetable shortening				

Conclusions:

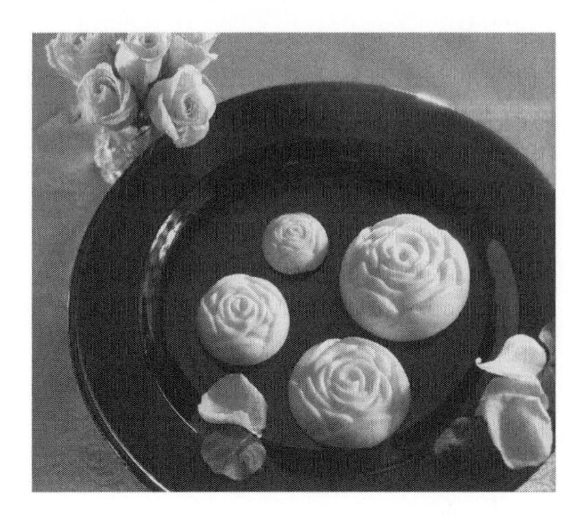

Butter Rosettes.
Courtesy: SYSCO® Incorporated.

SUMMARY QUESTIONS—FATS AND OILS

1. Define emulsion.

2. Define an emulsifier and how it functions.

3. When oil and vinegar are shaken together, which liquid is the continuous phase? Dispersed phase?

4. Distinguish between a temporary and permanent emulsion in an oil–vinegar mixture.

5. Identify food ingredients that have the potential to function as emulsifiers. List several processed foods that contain additives that function as emulsifiers (see Appendix E).

6. What constituent of eggs is the emulsifier?

7. What causes the emulsion in mayonnaise to break? How may the emulsion be re-formed?

8. Distinguish among French dressing, mayonnaise, and cooked dressing as to proportion of ingredients and the emulsifier used in preparation.

9. Other than salad dressing, which products prepared in class contain ingredients that emulsify the fat?

10. Explain why dressings for tossed salad should be added and mixed with the vegetables just before serving the salad.

11. Describe hydrogenation, noting the changes that occur in degree of saturation of the fats hydrogenated.

12. Which dietary fat is lowest in saturated fat? Which is highest?

13. Explain the role of fats in the human diet.

14. Concerning fat consumption in the United States: what is the average percentage of total calories coming from fat? What is the recommended percent?

15. Briefly list several ways Americans could lower their fat intake.

16. Identify several fat replacements and possible limitations with their use in foods.

17. Identify oils that contain known food allergens.

18. Identify several varieties of vinegar, used in preparing salad dressings with oil and vinegar, that contain known food allergens.

Dietitian's Note

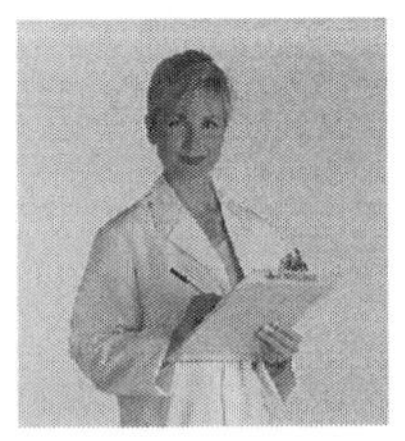

See websites listed under references.

Effective January 1, 2006 the FDA amended its regulations on nutrition labeling. Why is a declaration of trans fatty acids in the nutrition labeling of conventional foods and supplements required (21CFR Part 101)?

I. Sugars, Sweeteners

Taste and see that the Lord is good.

— Psalm 34:8

Objectives

To describe conditions prerequisite to crystallization of sugar solutions
To know and describe factors affecting the rate of crystallization and size of crystals in sugar products
To describe the relationship between boiling temperature, sugar concentration, and structure of sugar products
To describe and relate the effect of interfering agents to the structure of sugar products
To summarize key principles essential to obtaining a desirable sugar product
To demonstrate an understanding of and ability to apply key principles in the preparation of a sugar product
To evaluate the nutritive value of sugar products
To evaluate the uses and nutritive value of sugar substitutes
To discuss for whom a low-sugar diet is advantageous

References

http://www.sugar.org/
http://www.ussugar.com/

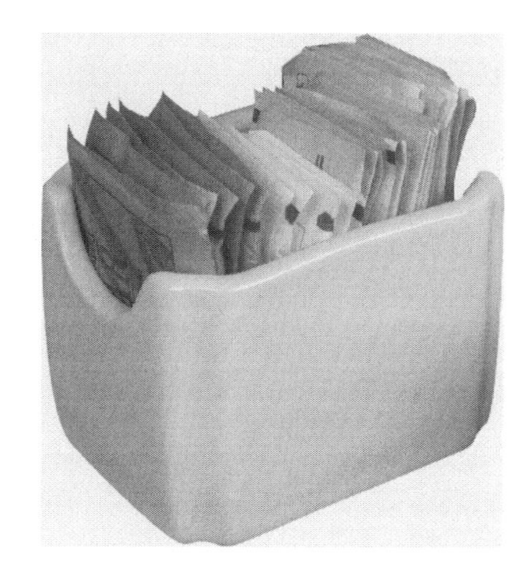

Sugar Sweeteners.
Courtesy: SYSCO® Incorporated.

Terms

Alternative sweeteners:
- Artificial sweeteners
- Sugar replacers

Amorphous
Caramelization
Crystalline
Crystallization
Heat of crystallization
Hydrolysis
Interfering agent
Inversion/invert sugar
Negative heat of solution
Nuclei
Saturated
Seeding
Solute
Solution
Solvent
Stevia
Supersaturated
Viscosity

CAUTION — SUGAR SYRUPS BURN!

EXERCISE 1: METHODS OF INITIATING CRYSTALLIZATION[1]

Procedure

Carry out or observe a demonstration of crystallization (requires overnight refrigeration).

1. Prepare a highly concentrated solution of sodium (Na) thiosulfate by adding 260 g sodium thiosulfate crystals to 100 mL boiling water. Stir to dissolve.
2. Pour into three similar sized beakers or other glass containers. Mark samples, cover, and refrigerate, undisturbed, overnight.
3. Carefully remove containers from refrigerator (the solutions are now supersaturated).
4. Initiate crystallization in the manner indicated below in the chart.

Method of Initiating Crystallization	Observations on Speed of Crystallization and Size of Crystal
Add 1 crystal of Na thiosulfate. Leave beaker undisturbed.	
Add 1 crystal of Na thiosulfate. Shake beaker vigorously.	
No addition of Na thiosulfate. Shake beaker vigorously.	

[1] Adapted from Halliday E.G. and I.T. Noble. 1943. *Food Chemistry and Cooking*. Chicago: University of Chicago Press.

1. Why was the solution cooled before crystallization was initiated?

2. What type of solution is necessary for crystallization to occur? Why?

3. Define the term *seeding*.

4. Does seeding affect crystal size? Why?

5. Does agitation affect crystal size? Why?

EXERCISE 2: THE RELATIONSHIP OF SUGAR CONCENTRATION TO BOILING POINT

PROCEDURE

1. Calibrate a thermometer.
2. Prepare proportions of sugar and water as directed.
3. Heat the mixtures in saucepans until boiling. Record the initial boiling point for each sample.
4. Continue boiling each solution to a temperature of 11°F (6°C) above the boiling point of water.
5. Immediately remove the solutions from heat. Cool slightly.
6. Using a glass measuring cup, measure the volume of each sugar solution. Record volumes. Reserve solutions for Exercise 3.

Water	Sugar	Initial Boiling Temperature	Final Boiling Temperature	Final Volume
A. 1 cup (240 ml)	½ cup (120 mL)			
B. ½ cup (120 mL)	½ cup (120 mL)			

1. How do the initial volumes of the sugar solutions compare?

2. How do the initial *boiling points* compare? Why?

3. How do the final volumes of the solutions compare? Why?

4. Why does solution A take longer to reach the specified final boiling point?

5. Based on this experiment, are the final concentrations of the sample the same or different? Explain.

EXERCISE 3: EFFECT OF TEMPERATURE AND AGITATION ON CRYSTAL SIZE

PROCEDURE

1. In a large saucepan mix 2 cups (480 mL) sugar and 1 cup (240 mL) hot water with the hot sugar syrups from Exercise 2.
2. Bring the mixture to a boil. Cover for a few minutes. Remove the cover and continue boiling without stirring.
3. When the solution reaches 236°F (113.5°C), remove saucepan from heat and divide the solution into approximately three parts as follows:
   a. Pour one-third over a thermometer placed on a marble slab. Cool undisturbed to 110°F (43.5°C). Manipulate with broad spatula until crystallization occurs. Knead until soft; then shape into patties.
   b. Pour one-third into another saucepan and immediately begin beating with a wooden spoon. Beat until crystallization occurs.
   c. Continue heating remaining third to 300°F (149°C). Immediately pour onto foil, making small wafer shapes.

Temperature When Agitated	Texture (e.g., Grainy/Smooth)	Appearance (e.g., Color/Shininess)
A. 110°F (43.5°C)		
B. Beaten immediately		
C. 300°F (149°C)		

1. Why were the crystal structures in A and B different? Describe the structures and account for the differences.

2. What was the final structure of C? Why did it differ from A and B?

3. Define "heat of crystallization." Was this observed in the experiments? If so, when?

EXERCISE 4: EFFECT OF INTERFERING AGENTS ON SUGAR STRUCTURE

Procedure

1. Calibrate a thermometer.
2. Prepare assigned recipes for crystalline or amorphous product. Circle interfering agents.
3. Display and evaluate all products. Note differences in structure.

PALATABILITY STANDARD	
AMORPHOUS	CRYSTALLINE
Caramels: smooth texture, no graininess, chewy, not sticky	Glossy
Brittle: smooth, hard	Smooth, creamy texture
Butterscotch: hard, clear amber color	Holds shape, yet soft

Candy Recipes[2]

Ingredients			Method
Old-Fashioned Butterscotch			
brown sugar	1 cup	240 mL	1. Combine first three ingredients. Bring to a boil.
light corn syrup	2 tbsp	30 mL	2. Cover pan for a few minutes. Uncover.
water	½ cup	120 mL	3. Cook, stirring as little as possible, to 288°F (142°C).
margarine/butter	2 tbsp	30 mL	4. Remove from heat. Stir in fat.
			5. Drop by teaspoonfuls on greased foil.

(continued on next page)

[2] Recipes may contain known allergens. See Appendix E.

Candy Recipes			
Ingredients			Method
Fondant			
sugar	1 cup	240 mL	1. Combine first three ingredients in a saucepan. Bring to a boil.
water	½ cup	120 mL	2. Cover pan for a few minutes.
cream of tartar	⅛ tsp	0.63 mL	3. Boil to 236°F (113.5°C) in uncovered pan.
flavoring	⅛ tsp	0.63 mL	4. Pour on marble slab.
			5. Add flavoring, cool undisturbed to 110°F (43.5°C).
			6. Beat until firm.
Chocolate Fudge			
sugar	1 cup	240 mL	1. Combine first four ingredients in a saucepan. Bring to a boil.
milk	⅜ cup	75 mL	
corn syrup	1 tbsp	15 mL	2. Cover pan for a few minutes.
chocolate square,	1 oz.	28 g	3. Boil to 234°F (112°C) in uncovered pan.
unsweetened	1 tbsp	15 mL	4. Remove from heat. Pour onto marble slab. Add fat and vanilla. Do not mix.
margarine/butter	½ tsp	2.5 mL	
vanilla			5. Cool, undisturbed, to 120°F (43.5°C).
			6. Beat until thick and creamy.
			7. Pour into greased 6-inch (15-cm) pan.
Peanut Brittle			
sugar	1 cup	240 mL	1. Combine first three ingredients. Bring to a boil.
light corn syrup	½ cup	120 mL	2. Cover pan for a few minutes. Uncover.
water	2 tbsp	30 mL	3. Heat to 238°F (114°C) stirring as little as possible.
margarine/butter	1½	22.5 mL	4. Add fat and peanuts. Stir constantly until 295°F (147°C).
peanuts	tbsp	120 mL	
vanilla	½ cup	2.5 mL	5. Add vanilla and soda. Stir.
baking soda	½ tsp	5 mL	6. Pour onto lightly greased foil, spreading syrup thin, but minimally.
	1 tsp		
Peanut Brittle, Microwave			
sugar	1 cup	240 mL	1. Combine first two ingredients. Microwave 3 minutes on HIGH in a glass bowl.
light corn syrup	½ cup	120 mL	
peanuts, unsalted	1 cup	240 mL	2. Add nuts and stir. Microwave on HIGH for 4 minutes.
margarine/butter	1 tsp	5 mL	3. Add fat, vanilla, and soda. Microwave on HIGH 1–2 minutes.
vanilla	1 tsp	5 mL	
baking soda	1 tsp	5 mL	4. Pour onto lightly greased foil, spreading syrup thin, but minimally. Cool at room temperature. Crack.

(continued on next page)

CANDY RECIPES

Ingredients			Method
Vanilla Caramels			
sugar	½ cup	120 mL	1. Combine all sugars and milk. Bring to a boil.
brown sugar	¼ cup	60 mL	2. Cover pan for a few minutes. Uncover.
light corn syrup	¼ cup	60 mL	3. Boil, stirring with a wooden spoon, to 240°F (116°C).
milk	½ cup	120 mL	4. Add evaporated milk and continue boiling until 248°F (120°C).
evaporated milk	¼ cup	60 mL	
margarine/butter	2 tbsp	30 mL	5. Remove from heat. Stir in fat and vanilla.
vanilla	½ tsp	2.5 mL	6. Pour into greased 6-inch (15-cm) pan.
Chocolate Fudge, Microwave			
sugar, confectioner's	1 lb.	454 g	1. Sift first two ingredients in a shallow, greased square glass pan. Stir in milk and pieces of cut margarine.
cocoa powder	½ cup	120 mL	
milk	¼ cup	60 mL	2. Microwave 2 minutes on HIGH. Add vanilla.
margarine	¼ lb.	115 g	3. Stir to blend.
vanilla	1 tbsp	15 mL	4. Refrigerate 1 hour. Cut into small square portions.

1. Compare the color and texture of fondant with that of the crystalline product in Exercise 3A. Account for the differences.

2. Compare the following interfering agents, noting how they foster small crystals in crystalline products or prevent crystallization in amorphous products.

Margarine/butter	
Milk	
Corn syrup	

3. How does the addition of baking soda contribute to the palatability of peanut brittle?

EXERCISE 5: ALTERNATIVES TO SUGAR[3]

Procedure

1. Study labels of several noncaloric artificial sweeteners and other alternatives to sugar and record ingredients below.
2. Evaluate the palatability of common sugar substitutes, in solution, comparing initial and aftertaste with sweetness of standard sugar solution. Record observations in the table.

Sweetener	Label Ingredients	Sweetener/1 cup (240 mL) water	Kcal/ solution	Initial Taste	Aftertaste
Standard		2 tsp sugar			
Acesulfame K		1 packet Sweet-One®			
Aspartame		1 packet Equal®			
Fructose		2 packets			
Sucralose		1 packet Splenda®			
Saccharin		1 packet Sweet 'N Low®			
Stevia		1 packet Truvia® (Rebiana™)			

1. Based on readings, list the current regulations that govern the use of these sugar substitutes in food products.

2. Identify nutritive (caloric) sugar alcohols and noncaloric or high-intensity sweeteners that are used in food products, noting specific products.

[3] Alternatives to sugar include the artificial sweeteners, which are high intensity and nonnutritive, and the sugar replacers/ sugar alcohols, which are caloric.

SUMMARY QUESTIONS—SUGARS, SWEETENERS

1. Why is a burn from boiling sugar syrup more severe than a burn from boiling water? Explain.

2. List important factors, common to all crystalline candy recipes, that influence the formation of small crystals.

3. As an uncovered sugar solution boils, why does the observed boiling point continue to rise? How does viscosity change?

4. In a fudge recipe, if the sugar is increased but the amount of liquids remains the same, how will the cooking time be affected?

5. In fudge preparation, if the end boiling point has been exceeded by 39°F (4°C), how can the product be corrected? Why is this possible?

6. In the preparation of peanut brittle, if the temperature exceeds 300°F (150°C) and a brownish-black mixture develops, can the product be corrected? Explain.

7. Identify several chemical interfering agents.

8. This graph illustrates the effect of interfering agents on the speed of crystallization of a sucrose solution.

   a. What is the effect of an interfering agent on the speed of crystallization?

   b. Why is a somewhat slower rate of crystallization helpful in keeping crystals small?

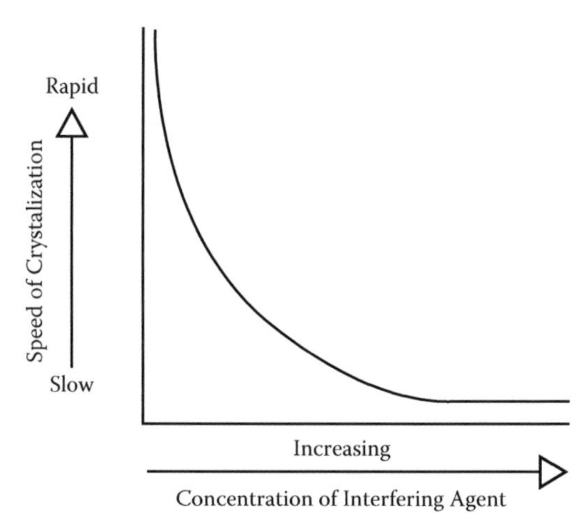

Source: Division of Nutritional Sciences, New York State College of Human Ecology at Cornell, Ithaca, New York.

9. Applying the principles of crystallization to the preparation of ice cream (freezing), predict how the following variables would affect crystal size.

Variable	Crystal Size
Slow rate of freezing	
No agitation	
Low freezing temperature	
Substitution of cream for milk	

10. In candy preparation, fudge fails to harden, and the texture is unsatisfactory. How might a new brand of sugar, 51% sucrose and 49% fructose, be the cause of this product failure? Would the results have been unsatisfactory if this sugar had been used in the preparation of peanut brittle?

11. Discuss why artificial sweeteners/sugar substitutes may not be effective in all prepared foods as a major ingredient. What precautions must be observed?

12. Identify advantages and disadvantages of using sugar substitutes, considering cost, function, and nutritive value.

13. Identify sugar substitute, reduced-sugar, or sugar-free products that also use fat substitute, reduced-fat, or fat-free formulations. Identify advantages and disadvantages of using these products.

14. Discuss the benefits of a low-sugar way of eating.

Dietitian's Note

Categories of alternatives to table sugar:

1. **Artificial sweeteners/sugar substitutes**—FDA approved: saccharin, aspartame, acesulfame potassium (acesulfame K), sucralose, neotame. Noncaloric because they provide no energy. Also called nonnutritive.

2. **Sugar replacers/sugar alcohols**—mannitol, sorbitol, xylitol, malitol, isomalt. Caloric. Sugar-free does not indicate calorie-free. Despite the name, the sugar alcohols contain neither sugar nor alcohol.

3. **Other natural sweeteners**—including stevia, a zero-calorie sweetener from the leaves of the *Stevia* plant; Rebiana is a trade name; Truvia® is the consumer brand.

J. Batters and Dough

Man shall not live by bread alone.

— Deuteronomy 8:3

Objectives

To describe the function of ingredients in a variety of products made from batters and doughs
To compare the gluten potential of flours made from wheat, corn, rye, and soy
To assess the effectiveness of different leavening agents and relate these to palatability characteristics
To delineate relationships of kind and proportion of ingredients to final product characteristics
To evaluate the effect of manipulation on gluten development in a variety of batters and doughs
To relate gluten development to palatability characteristics of products made from various batters and dough
To distinguish palatability characteristics such as flakiness, tenderness, and grain in batters and dough
To compare subjective and objective measurements in assessing palatability of pastry
To evaluate nutritive value of different grains
To identify food allergens and acceptable recipe alternatives in baked goods.

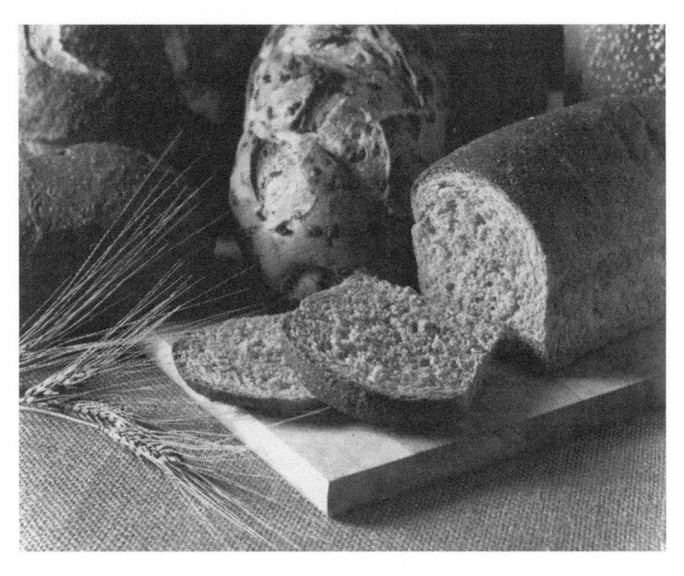

Whole Wheat Bread.
Source: Division of Nutritional Sciences, New York State College of Human Ecology at Cornell, Ithaca, New York.

References

Appendices E, L, N
www.MyPyramid.com
www.grainpower.org
www.wheatfoods.org
http://www.ncaur.usda.gov/cpf/trimtech.html
http://www.celiac.com
www.csaceliacs.org; search Gluten free diet; Celiac Sprue Association
http://www.gluten.net

Terms

All-purpose flour
Cell size
Cell walls
Cohesive
Conventional method
Cornmeal
Cream
Crumbs
Dump method
Egg allergy
Elastic
Emulsifier
Fermentation
Flakiness
Fold
Food allergen
Gluten development
Gluten-free
Gluten potential
Grain
Hydration
Hydrogenated fat
Knead
Lactose intolerance
Leavening
Legume allergy
Milk protein allergy
Muffin method
Nut allergy
Oven spring
Pastry method
Peaks
Plastic fat
Rice flour
Rye flour
Saturated fat
Soy flour
Tenderness
Tunnels
Unsaturated fat
Whole grain/whole wheat flour

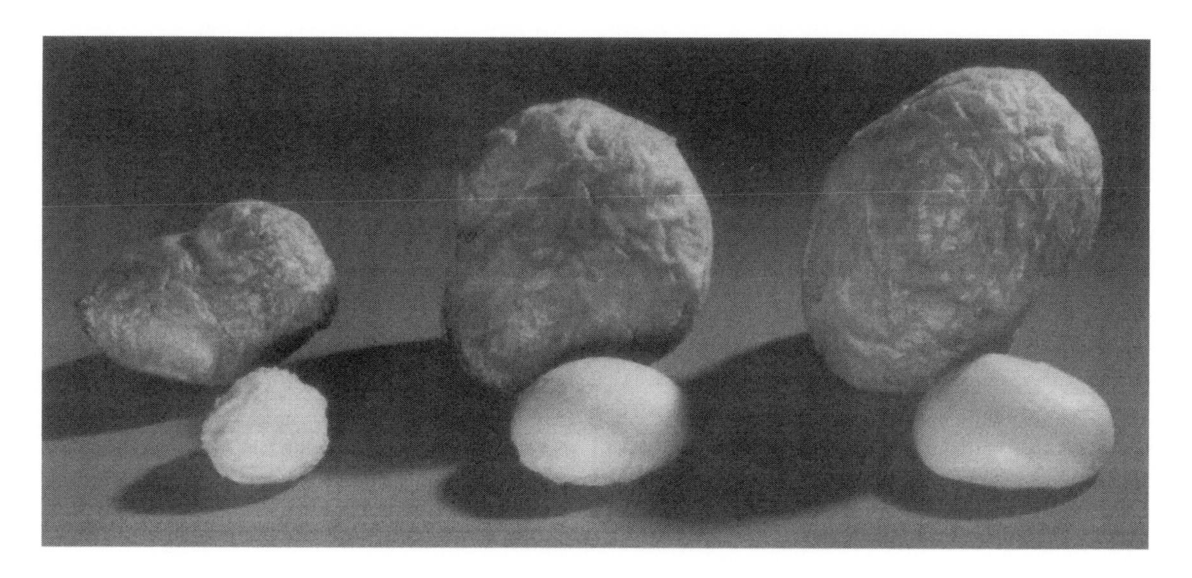

Gluten Balls, Unbaked and Baked. (Left to Right): Cake Flour, All-Purpose Flour, and Bread Flour.
Courtesy: Wheat Flour Institute.

EXERCISE 1: MEASUREMENT OF FLOUR

Procedure

1 a. Weigh 1 cup (240 mL) ***unsifted*** all-purpose flour as directed on chart.
1 b. Sift flour. Gently scoop 1 cup (240 mL) of ***sifted*** flour into measuring cup without packing. Level off with straight-edge knife and weigh only what fits in 1 cup.
2. Compare results of the two weights with classmates and account for differences.

	Weight (g)	Class Range and Average (g)
Unsifted flour		
Sifted flour		

Why are there differences in weight between unsifted and sifted flour?

EXERCISE 2: STRUCTURAL PROPERTIES OF WHEAT FLOUR

Procedure

Either prepare or observe a demonstration of making gluten balls as follows:

1. Mix 1 cup (240 mL) all-purpose flour with approximately ¼ cup (60 mL) water until all of the water is absorbed.
2. Knead dough 10 to 15 minutes until it is cohesive and elastic.

3. Place dough in a bowl filled with cold water; squeeze the dough to work out the starch. Repeat the process with fresh water until the bowl water is clear.
4. Press water from the dough. Bake dough ball at 400°F (205°C) for about 30 minutes, until firm.

QUESTIONS—GLUTEN[1]

1. Why is cold water used to remove the starch?

2. As flour and cold water are mixed to make a dough, what is happening to the starch component of the flour?

3. As the dough is kneaded, what is happening to the protein in the flour?

4. How does the baked gluten ball differ from the unbaked?

[1] Gluten is a known allergen. See Appendix E.

5. What is the source of leavening in gluten balls?

6. What is meant by the gluten potential of a flour?

7. Why are gluten balls from cake flour, all-purpose flour, and bread flour different in size?

8. How do the wheat flour gluten balls compare to those attempted with use of a low gluten potential flour? A non-gluten flour? Explain.

EXERCISE 3: CHEMICAL LEAVENING AGENTS

A. Ingredients of Baking Powders

Procedure

1. Inspect labels on several baking powder cans.
2. Complete the following chart.

Baking Powder	Alkali	Acid	Teaspoons/Cup Flour (mL/240 mL)

B. Comparison of Speed of Reaction

Procedure

1. Mix 1 tsp (5 mL) specified leavening with liquid (1 tbsp [15 mL]) as directed.
2. Observe the speed of reaction.
3. Summarize conclusions about speed of reaction and ingredients.

Leavening	Liquid	Relative Speed of Gas Production
Baking soda	1 tbsp cold water	
Baking soda	1 tbsp hot water	
Baking soda	1 tbsp vinegar	
Baking soda + ¼ tsp (1.25 mL) cream of tartar	1 tbsp cold water	
Tartrate baking powder	1 tbsp cold water	
Double-acting baking powder	1 tbsp cold water	
Double-acting baking powder	1 tbsp hot water	

Conclusions:

EXERCISE 4: FACTORS AFFECTING THE LEAVENING POWER OF YEAST

Procedure

1. Prepare standard mixture as follows for each of three small custard cups:
   1 package dry yeast
      2 tbsp (30 mL) water, room temperature
      1 tbsp (15 mL) flour
      ¼ tsp (1.25 mL) sugar
2. Add the sugar and salt variables to the standard mixture as directed. Stir and allow all mixtures to react for 25 minutes.
3. Observe the rate of gas production and summarize results.

Variable	Rate of Gas Production
Standard	
Standard + 2 tbsp (30 mL) sugar	
Standard + 1 tsp (5 mL) salt	

Conclusions:

QUESTIONS—LEAVENING AGENTS

1. List some acid foods that are commonly used with baking soda.

2. To what components of baking powder do the terms "single-acting" and "double-acting" refer? Why are the terms accurate?

3. What is the role of starch in baking powders?

4. Account for the "soapy" taste in products that have excess soda.

5. Why are soda-acid-leavened products often extremely tender?

6. What environmental factors must be present to ensure adequate growth for yeast?

7. How does the leavening action of yeast differ from that of baking powder?

EXERCISE 5: DROP BATTERS, MUFFINS[2,3]

Basic Muffin Recipe

sifted all-purpose flour	1 cup	240 mL	egg	1	
sugar	2 tbsp	30 mL	milk	½ cup	120 mL
double-acting baking powder	1½ tsp	7.5 mL	oil	2 tbsp	30 mL

1. Grease six muffin cups (or use paper liners) and set oven at 425°F (220°C).
2. Sift the dry ingredients into a mixing bowl.
3. Beat the egg slightly, add milk and oil.
4. Make a well in the dry ingredients. Add the liquid ingredients and stir until the dry ingredients are just moistened (about 16 stirs). The batter will be lumpy.
5. Fill the greased muffin cups half-full.
6. Bake the muffins about 20 minutes, until golden brown.

A. Effect of Manipulation

Procedure

1. Follow the basic muffin recipe, using 16 stirs or until dry ingredients are just moistened. Then
   a. Place 2 portions (about ¼ cup, 80 mL) of batter in muffin pan.
   b. Stir remaining batter 5 additional strokes and remove 2 portions.
   c. Stir remaining batter 25 additional strokes and remove 2 portions. Bake 6 muffins.
2. Evaluate baked products on the chart.

[2] Refer to the chapter on Microwave Cooking for microwave recipes.
[3] Recipes may contain known allergens. Refer to Appendix E.

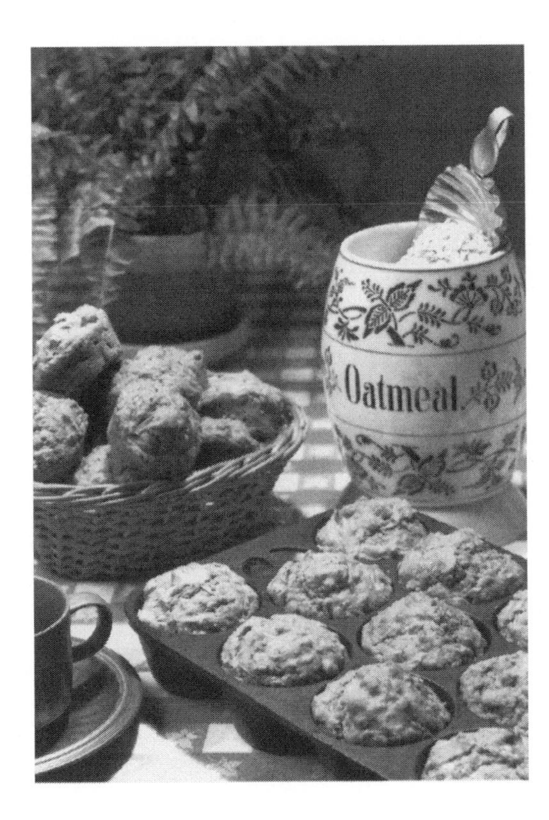

Oatmeal Muffins.
Source: Cornell University, Cooperative Extension, Ithaca, New York.

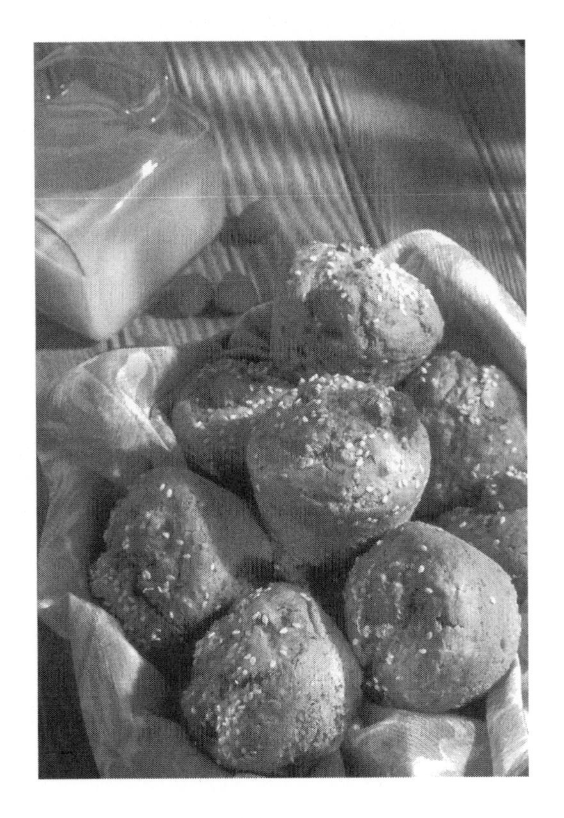

Muffins.
Courtesy: SYSCO® Incorporated.

3. Summarize the effects of manipulation on palatability (see chart) characteristics of muffins.

Characteristic	Amount of Manipulation		
	Mix until Moistened	Additional 5 Strokes	Additional 25 Strokes
Color			
Shape			
Volume			
Tenderness			
Grain (cell size, tunnels, etc.)			
Extent of gluten development			

Conclusion:

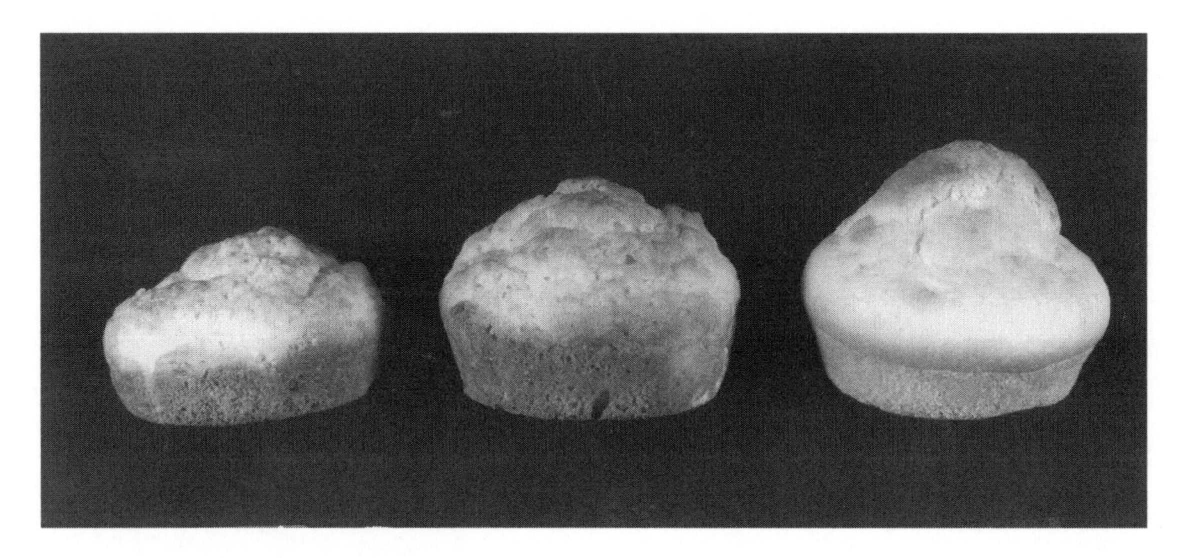

Effect of Manipulation on Muffins: (left to right) Undermixed, Mixed to Moisten, and Overmixed.

Source: Division of Nutritional Sciences, New York State College of Human Ecology at Cornell, Ithaca, New York.

PALATABILITY STANDARD—MUFFINS

APPEARANCE	TEXTURE OF CRUMB	TENDERNESS
Volume: double unbaked	Uniform	Breaks easily
Top: uneven, pebbled, slightly rounded golden brown	Air cell: medium-coarse Cell walls: medium thick	Soft in mouth

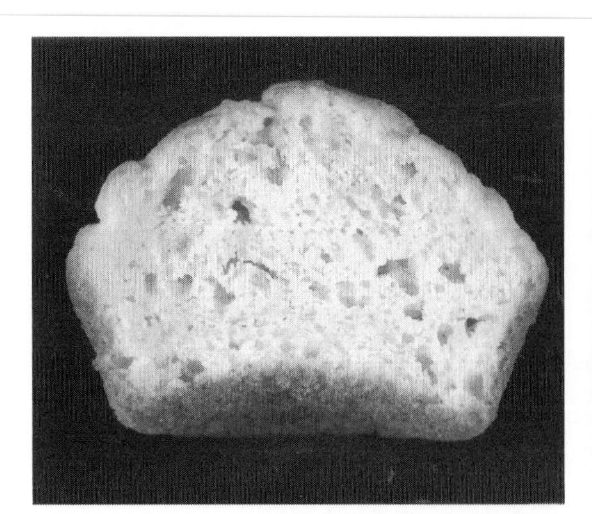

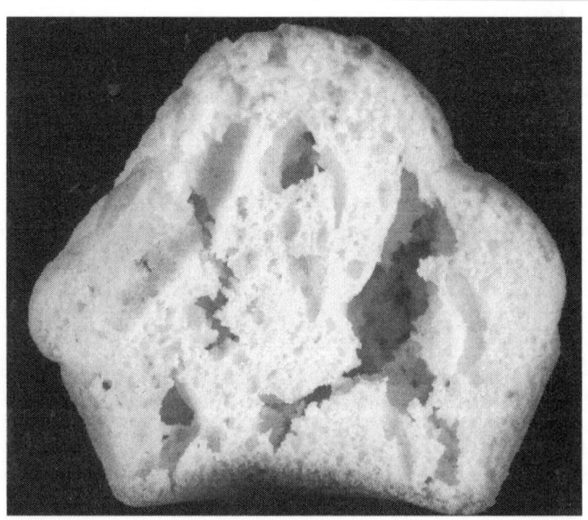

Correctly Mixed Batter (left): Muffin Has Rounded Top, Even Texture; (right): Overmixed Batter, Muffin Has Tunnels and Peak.

Source: Division of Nutritional Sciences, New York State College of Human Ecology at Cornell, Ithaca, New York.

B. Effect of Different Grains

Procedure

1. Follow the basic muffin recipe, substituting other flours, as directed (50/50 = half all-purpose, half designated flour type listed).
2. Evaluate all products on the following chart. Summarize results.

Flour	Volume	Texture	Tenderness of Crumb	Extent of Gluten Development
Cornmeal 100%				
50/50				
Whole wheat 100%				
50/50				
Rye 100%				
50/50				
Soy 50/50				
25% soy				
Rice 100%				
50/50				

QUESTIONS—MUFFINS

1. What is the ratio of liquid to flour in a muffin recipe? How does this ratio affect gluten development?

2. What are the sources of leavening in muffins?

3. Why do most muffin recipes specify liquid fat (oil or melted solid)? How does fat function in a muffin batter?

4. What causes tunnels? Were tunnels prevalent in muffins made with the cornmeal and whole wheat flour? Explain.

5. Why does wheat flour have a high gluten potential? Why are corn and rye low?

6. How may a desirable structure be obtained if low gluten potential flour (rye, cornmeal) is desired in a muffin recipe?

EXERCISE 6: SOFT DOUGH, BISCUITS[4,5]

Basic Biscuit Recipe

sifted all-purpose flour	2 cups	480 mL	fat, hydrogenated	¼ cup	60 mL
double-acting baking powder	1 tbsp	15 mL	milk	⅔ cup	160 mL

1. Set oven at 425°F (220°C).
2. Sift the dry ingredients into a mixing bowl.
3. Cut the fat into the dry ingredients, using a pastry blender or two knives, one in each hand. Continue cutting until no fat particles are larger than peas.
4. Add the milk and mix vigorously with a fork until the dough is stiff (about 25 times), cutting through the center of the dough with the fork several times.
5. Knead 10 times on lightly floured counter; roll to 1-inch (2.54-cm) thickness.
6. Cut to shape and bake 12 minutes or until brown.

---

[4] Refer to the chapter on Microwave Cooking for microwave recipes.
[5] Recipes may contain known allergens. Refer to Appendix E.

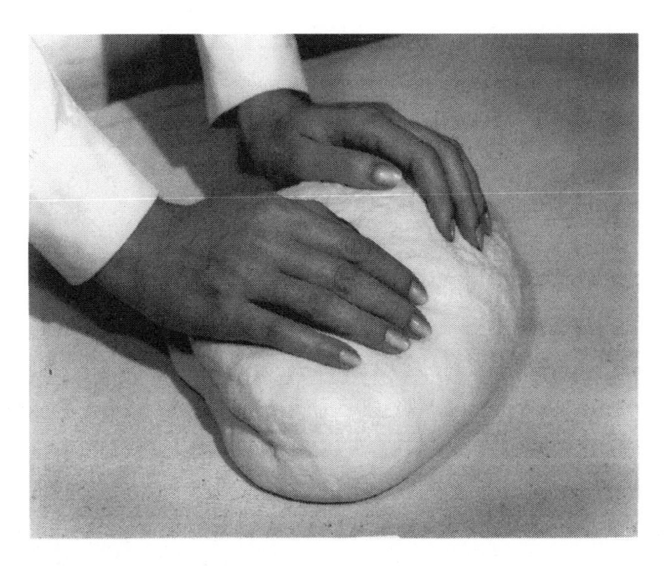

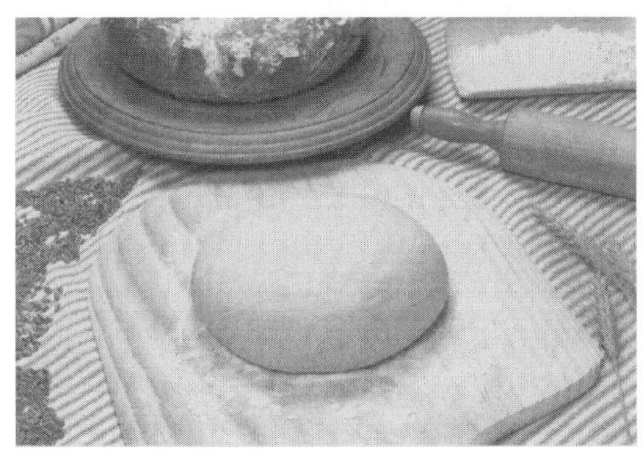

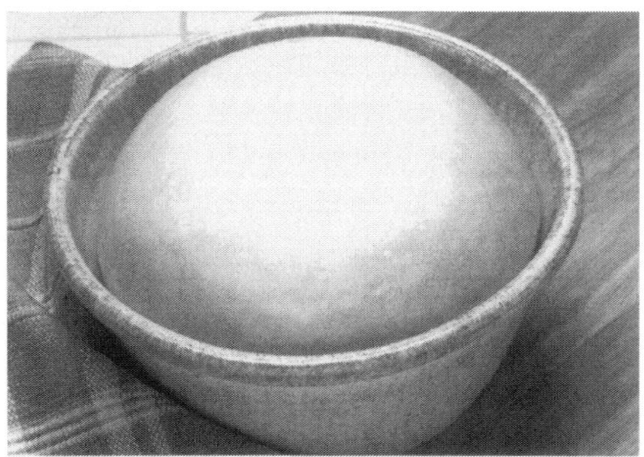

Kneading Dough.

Courtesy: Wheat Flour Institute (top). *Courtesy:* Wheat Foods Council (bottom left and right).

PALATABILITY STANDARD—BISCUITS

APPEARANCE	TEXTURE	TENDERNESS
Volume doubled	Uniform	Crust: crisp, easy to break
Top: golden brown, flat, circular	Air cell size: small	Crumb: soft to touch, moist
Sides: straight	Cell walls: thin	
	Flaky layers	

A. Effect of Manipulation

Procedure

1. Follow basic biscuit recipe through step 4.
2. Divide dough into three portions.
3. Lightly flour board and rolling pin.
4. Manipulate dough, kneading as directed. Roll to 1 inch (2.54 cm) thick.
5. Cut and bake for 12 minutes.
6. Evaluate products and summarize the effect of manipulation on palatability of the biscuits.
7. Save the biscuits that were kneaded 10 times (variation b) to use as the standard for Part B.

	Amount of Manipulation		
Palatability	No Kneading	Kneaded 10 Times	Kneaded 30 Times
Appearance			
Volume			
Shape			
Texture			
Cell size			
Flakiness			
Tenderness			
Extent of gluten development			

Conclusions:

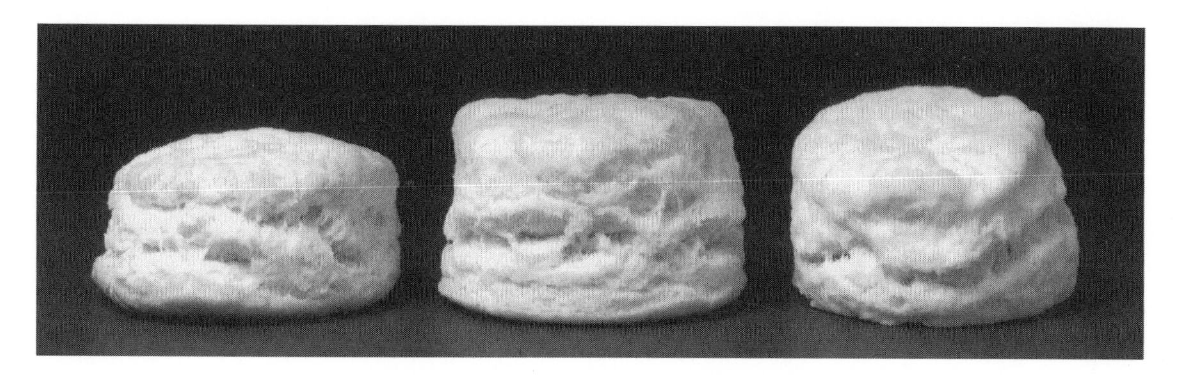

EFFECT OF MANIPULATION ON BISCUITS (LEFT TO RIGHT): NO KNEADING, KNEADED 10 TIMES, AND KNEADED EXTENSIVELY.
Source: Division of Nutritional Sciences, New York State College of Human Ecology at Cornell, Ithaca, New York.

B. SUBSTITUTING SODA ACID FOR BAKING POWDER

PROCEDURE

1. Follow the basic biscuit recipe, substituting 1 cup (160 mL) buttermilk for regular milk and using ½ tsp (2.5 mL) baking soda and 2 tsp (10 mL) double-acting baking powder as leavening.
2. Mix as directed and knead 10 times.
3. Cut and bake 12 minutes or until brown.
4. Evaluate products, comparing soda-acid biscuits with standard baking powder biscuits (in Part A, variation b). Record observations.

Palatability	Standard Baking Powder	Soda-Acid
Appearance Volume		
Shape		
Color of crust		
Texture Cell size		
Flakiness		
Tenderness		

QUESTIONS—BISCUITS

1. What is the ratio of liquid to flour in a biscuit recipe?

2. How does this ratio affect the development of gluten?

3. What are the sources of leavening in the biscuits?

4. How does fat function in a biscuit recipe?

5. How would the state of the fat (solid or liquid) affect the texture of a biscuit?

6. Based on the experiments, how do the palatability characteristics of a soda-acid biscuit differ from a biscuit leavened by baking powder?

7. In substituting soda for baking powder, what are the proportions used? What is the amount of soda used to neutralize 1 cup (240 mL) buttermilk or sour milk?

EXERCISE 7: PANCAKES, POPOVERS, CREAM PUFFS, CREPES

A. Effect of Manipulation on Gluten Development in Pancakes

Basic Pancake Recipe[6,7]

sifted all-purpose flour	1¼ cups	300 mL	egg	1	
baking powder	1¾ tsp	9 mL	milk	1 cup	240 mL
sugar	2 tbsp	30 mL	oil	2 tbsp	30 mL

1. Sift dry ingredients into medium bowl.
2. Beat wet ingredients and add to dry ingredients.
3. Stir quickly only until ingredients are combined; batter will be somewhat lumpy.
4. Bake on a hot griddle or heavy skillet until bubbles form on surface and edges become dry. Turn, cook approximately 2 minutes until golden brown.

---

[6] As a variation, use ½ cup (120 mL) whole wheat flour and ¾ cup (180 mL) all-purpose flour.

[7] Recipes may contain known allergens. Refer to Appendix E.

PALATABILITY STANDARD—PANCAKE		
APPEARANCE	TEXTURE	TENDERNESS
Volume: double unbaked	Uniform, even	Crust: easy to cut
Shape: regular	Air cell size: medium-fine	Crumb: light, moist, not gummy
Color: evenly browned	Cell walls: medium	

Procedure

1. Follow the basic recipe through step 2, but mix as follows:
   a. Stir liquid and dry ingredients only until moistened. Remove ½ cup (120 mL) batter and bake two pancakes.
   b. Stir remaining batter an additional 25 strokes and bake two pancakes.
2. Evaluate products and summarize results.

Palatability	Until Moistened	Additional 25 Strokes
Appearance		
Texture		
Tenderness		
Extent of gluten development		

Conclusions:

B. Effect of Manipulation on Gluten Development in Popovers

Basic Popover Recipe

flour, sifted	½ cup	120 mL	milk	½ cup	120 mL
egg	1				

1. Set oven at 425°F (220°C) and lightly grease four 5-oz. (150-mL) custard cups.
2. Sift flour into small bowl. Add egg and milk.
3. Beat with electric or rotary beater until smooth.
4. Pour into custard cups, place on baking sheet.
5. Bake for 40 to 45 minutes, or until golden brown, reducing oven temperature to 375°F (190°C) after 20 minutes.
6. Evaluate products and summarize results.

PALATABILITY STANDARD—POPOVER

APPEARANCE	TEXTURE
Volume: double or triple unbaked	Crust: crisp
Color: medium brown shiny crust	Inside: hollow, moist but not soggy, light, airy

PROCEDURE

1. Follow the basic popover recipe through step 3, then proceed as follows:
   a. Place half of the batter into two greased custard cups. Bake as directed.
   b. Beat the remaining batter an additional minute, and pour into two greased custard cups. Bake.
2. Compare products and summarize results using palatability standard provided.

Palatability	Beaten until Smooth	Beaten Additional 1 min
Appearance		
Texture		
Tenderness Crust		
Crumb		

Conclusions:

C. CREAM PUFFS

Basic Cream Puff Recipe

water	½ cup	120 mL	flour, sifted	½ cup	120 mL
margarine	¼ cup	60 mL	eggs, medium	2	

1. Set oven at 450°F (230°C) and lightly grease a baking sheet.
2. Place water and fat in a medium saucepan and bring to a boil to melt fat.
3. Immediately add all the flour and stir vigorously until the batter is smooth and forms a ball. Remove pan from the heat.
4. Add eggs, one at a time, beating well after each addition.
5. Drop batter into four mounds on baking sheet and bake for 15 minutes; reduce oven temperature to 350°F (175°C). Bake 20 minutes longer or until puffs are lightly brown and firm.
6. Evaluate products and summarize results.

PROCEDURE

1. Prepare cream puffs according to recipe.
2. Evaluate palatability of final product; account for any differences from Palatability Standard.

PALATABILITY STANDARD—CREAM PUFF		
APPEARANCE	TEXTURE	TENDERNESS
Volume: double unbaked	Hollow center, one large hole	Crust: crisp, tender
Shape: rounded		Interior: slightly moist
Color: golden brown		

Palatability	Reasons for Variations from Standard Product (if Applicable)
Appearance	
Texture	
Tenderness	

D. CREPES

Basic Crepe Recipe

butter/margarine, melted	1 tbsp	15 mL	egg yolk	1	
flour, sifted	1 cup	240 mL	milk (all may not be used)	1 cup	240 mL
eggs	1				

1. Sift flour into medium bowl.
2. Make a hole in the center and add melted butter and wet ingredients very slowly, incorporating all flour (less than 1 cup [240 mL] milk may be required).
3. Stir carefully until ingredients are combined; let rest in a cool place for 1 hour.
4. Using 2 to 3 tbsp (30 to 45 mL) for each crepe, fry each crepe on a hot crepe pan, for 1½ minutes on the first side. Turn, cook approximately 1 minute until golden brown.
5. Store crepes between layers of wax paper (crepes may be prepared ahead of time and filled with a sweet or savory filling).
6. Evaluate appearance, texture, and flavor.

PROCEDURE

1. Follow recipe.
2. Evaluate products according to appearance, texture, and flavor.

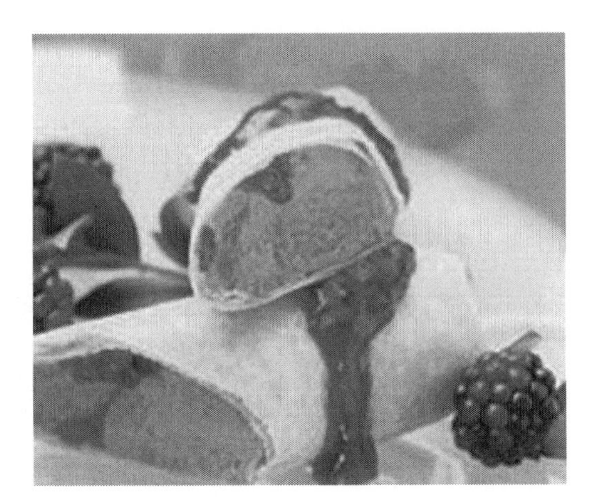

CREPES.
Courtesy: SYSCO® Incorporated.

EVALUATION OF CREPES

	Evaluation
Appearance	
Texture	
Tenderness	

QUESTIONS—PANCAKES, POPOVERS, CREAM PUFFS, CREPES

1. What is the proportion of liquid to flour in pancakes and popovers? What effect does this proportion have on the development of gluten?

2. How are pancakes leavened? How are popovers leavened?

3. Predict the effect on palatability if pancakes are turned after bubbles burst. What are the bubbles?

4. Why is a high initial oven temperature essential to the leavening of popovers and cream puffs?

5. In addition to contributing to structure, how does the egg function in the cream puff dough?

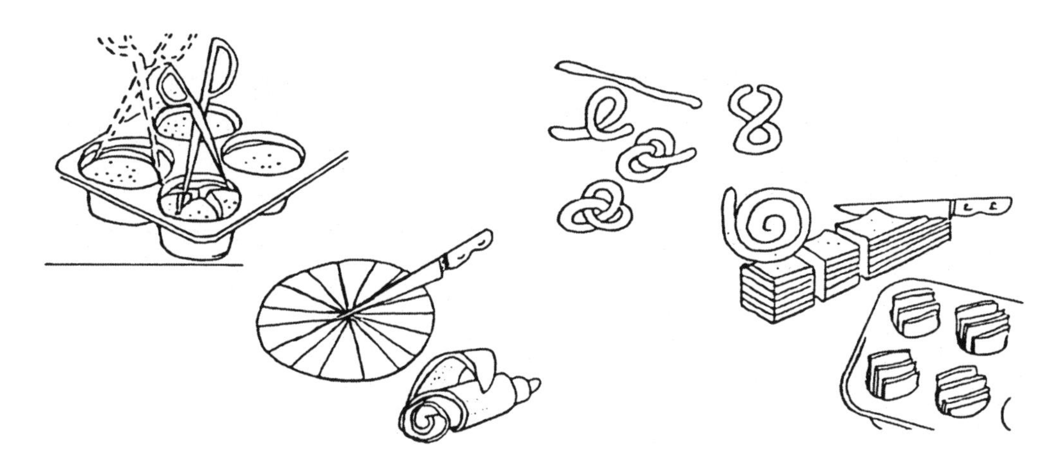

Shaping Yeast Dough.
Courtesy: USDA.

EXERCISE 8: STIFF DOUGH—YEAST BREADS/ROLLS

Procedure

1. Prepare yeast rolls according to the recipe below.
2. Evaluate final product. Does the product differ from the Palatability Standard. If so, explain.

Yeast Rolls

water, warm	⅔ cup	60 mL	salt[a]	1 tsp	5 mL
dry yeast[b]	½–1 package		flour[c]	2½–3 cups	600–720 mL
sugar	2 tbsp	30 mL	egg (optional)	1	
nonfat dry milk solids	⅓ cup	80 mL	vegetable oil	2 tbsp	30 mL

[a] Salt is a required ingredient because it regulates the growth of yeast.
[b] If laboratory time is short, use 1 package yeast.
[c] Up to half of the flour can be whole wheat.

1. Place warm water (105°F to 115°F, 40°C to 46°C) in a large mixing bowl.
2. Stir the dry yeast and sugar into the water.
3. Add the milk and salt to the yeast–water mixture.
4. Stir in the flour, 1 cup (240 mL) at a time, alternating with the eggs and oil. Beat well after each addition.
5. Add enough of the remaining flour to make a soft dough.
6. Turn dough onto a well-floured board and knead until smooth and elastic. The dough will spring back when touched.
7. Place dough in slightly oiled bowl; oil the top of the dough, cover tightly.
8. Allow to double in volume at room temperature. Dough has risen sufficiently if pressed finger marks remain in the dough.
9. Punch dough down and knead until smooth and elastic on an unfloured (or lightly floured) board.

10. Shape the dough into desired type of rolls (see illustration, Shaping Yeast Dough).
11. Place the rolls on a lightly greased pan and brush with oil. Set oven at 400°F (205°C).
12. Allow rolls to double in volume (about 45 minutes on counter.
13. Bake for 10 to 15 minutes, or until browned (20 medium rolls).
14. Evaluate products and summarize results.

PALATABILITY STANDARD—YEAST ROLLS			
APPEARANCE	**TEXTURE**	**TENDERNESS**	**FLAVOR**
Symmetrical	Uniform	Crust: thin, easy to cut	Fresh
Crust: golden smooth	Air cells: medium-fine	Crumb: silky, moist	Not yeasty
Volume: doubled	Cell walls: thin		Not flat

EVALUATION OF YEAST ROLLS

	Reasons for Variation from Standard Product (if Applicable)
Appearance	
Shape	
Volume	
Texture	
Uniformity	
Cell size	
Cell walls	
Tenderness	
Crust	
Crumb	
Flavor	

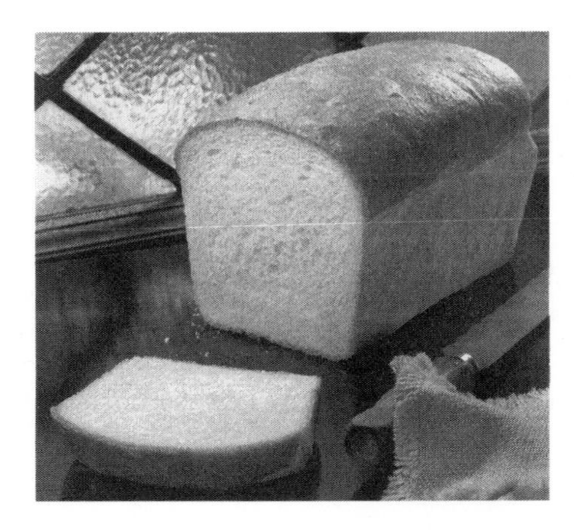

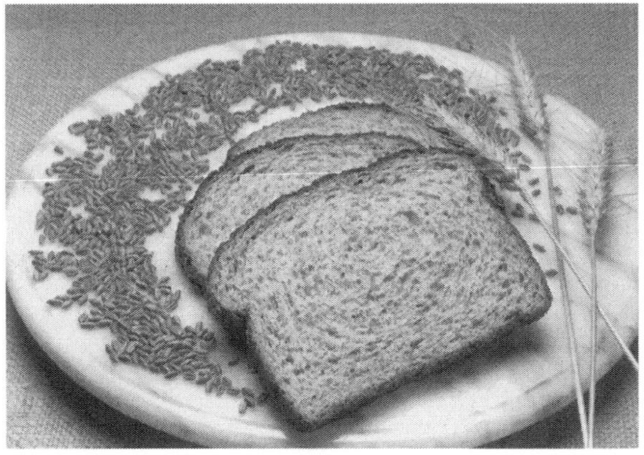

YEAST BREAD (LEFT); CRACKED WHEAT BREAD (RIGHT).
NOTE EXCELLENT VOLUME, UNIFORM TEXTURE, AND MEDIUM-SIZED AIR CELLS.
Courtesy: USDA (left) and Wheat Foods Council (right).

QUESTIONS—YEAST BREADS/ROLLS

1. What is the ratio of liquid to flour in yeast dough? How does this ratio affect gluten development?

2. List the products of yeast dough fermentation and state how each affects the quality of the baked product.

3. Explain why extensive gluten development is advantageous in yeast-leavened products.

4. List the ingredients that are essential for bread making. Explain.

5. Is it necessary to scald milk(s) for addition in a bread recipe? At what temperature should fluid milk be, before combining it with yeast? Why? How may milk temperature be determined without use of a thermometer?

6. What are the effects of allowing yeast to rise too much? Too little?

7. What is meant by "oven spring"?

8. Predict the relative volume of a sweet yeast dough compared to the yeast-roll recipe used in the laboratory.

9. Identify what happens to the ingredients in yeast rolls during the following processes:

Process	Flour	Liquid	Yeast	Sugar
Mixing				
Kneading				
Rising				
Baking				

EXERCISE 9: SHORTENED CAKES

A. Effect of Manipulation and Type of Shortening on Cake Texture

Procedure

1. Prepare a cake using assigned method of mixing and assigned shortening.
2. Evaluate batter characteristics and palatability characteristics of all variables. Record observations.

Shortened Cake[8]

shortening	⅓ cup	80 mL	sifted cake flour or	1 cup	240 mL
vanilla	½ tsp	2.5 mL	all-purpose flour	½ cup	120 mL
sugar	⅔ cup	160 mL	double-acting baking powder	1 tsp	5 mL
eggs	1½		milk	⅓ cup	80 mL

[8] Use butter, margarine, or hydrogenated fat. You may experiment with a fat-free spread.

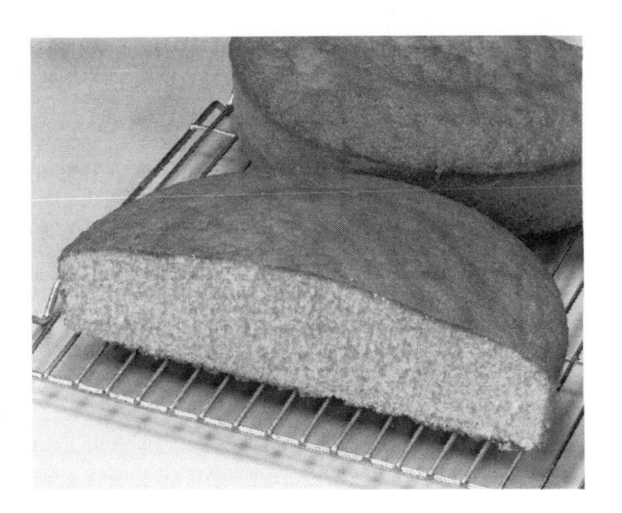

Conventional cake. Note excellent volume, uniform texture, and thin cell walls.
Courtesy: General Mills.

CONVENTIONAL METHOD OF MIXING

1. Set oven at 350°F (175°C) and grease 6-inch (15-cm) or larger pans.
2. Add vanilla to assigned shortening and cream until soft.
3. Gradually add sugar to softened fat and cream until light and fluffy using hand mixer set on medium speed. (Mixing by hand: add 2 tbsp (30 mL) of sugar at a time and beat 100 strokes after each addition.)
4. Add unbeaten eggs, mixing until blended (150 strokes by hand).
5. Sift dry ingredients. Add dry ingredients alternately with milk, beginning and ending with flour. Mix just until a smooth batter is formed.
6. Pour batter into prepared pan. Bake for 30 minutes, or until a toothpick inserted into cake comes out clean.
7. Set cake on rack and cool 10 minutes before removing the cake from the pan.

DUMP METHOD OF MIXING

1. Sift dry ingredients into a large bowl.
2. Add wet ingredients.
3. Beat batter with hand mixer set on medium speed, for 2 minutes, cleaning sides of bowl. Beat for 2 additional minutes.
4. Pour batter into prepared pan and proceed as directed for conventional cake.

EVALUATION OF CAKES

Shortening	Appearance	Texture	Mouthfeel
Butter Conventional			
Dump Method			
Margarine Conventional			
Dump			
Hydrogenated fat Conventional			
Dump			

Conclusions:

PALATABILITY STANDARD—CAKE

APPEARANCE	TEXTURE OF CRUMB	MOUTHFEEL
Volume: double unbaked	Uniform	Slightly moist
Top: slightly rounded, golden brown	Air cell size: small–medium	Velvety
	Cell walls: thin	Light

QUESTIONS—CAKES

1. In the conventional method of mixing, what is the purpose of creaming?

2. What is the function of eggs in shortened cakes?

3. Which assigned shortening contained an emulsifier? What is an emulsifier, and how does it act to improve the cake quality?

4. Why atition to fat, what other ingredients influence volume and texture of the cake?

5. In addition to fat, what other ingredients influence volume and texture of the cake?

EXERCISE 10: STIFF DOUGH—PASTRY

A. Effect of Different Fat Plasticities on Palatability of Pastry[9,10]

Procedure

1. Follow the basic pastry recipe to prepare a one-crust pie shell using assigned shortening (at room or refrigerator temperature).
2. Evaluate all variables and record evaluations using the letter corresponding to the appropriate term.
3. Summarize the relationship between type of shortening and subjective measurements of palatability.
4. After evaluation, choose one fat to bake pastry for assigned pie.[10]

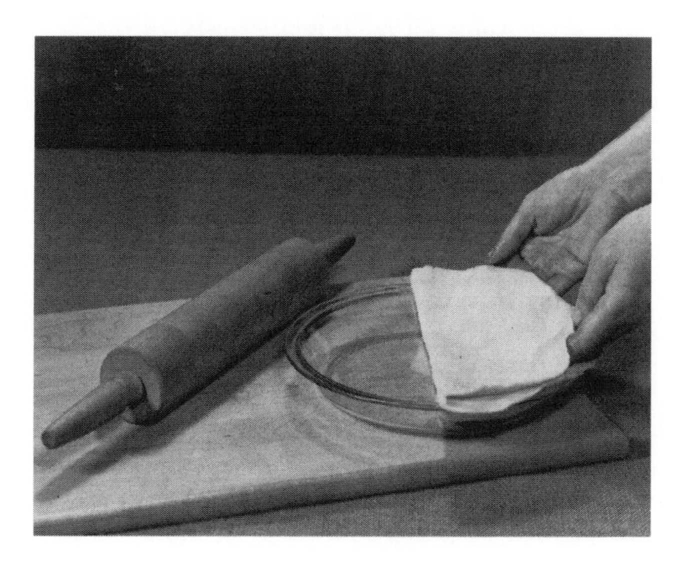

Placing Crust in Pie Plate.
Courtesy: General Mills.

[9] May be completed in the chapter on Fats and Oils, utilizing various fats and oils, and fat-free spreads.
[10] After experimentation using various fats, try one of the recipes using a premade pie crust. A premade crust may require only unfolding or unrolling prior to filling and baking.

Basic Pastry Recipe

flour, sifted	¾ cup	180 mL	shortening (fat or oil)	¼ cup	60 mL
water	1 tbsp + 2 tsp	25 mL			

1. Set oven at 375°F (190°C).
2. Cut solid fat into the flour until the largest particles are about the size of peas.
3. Add the water and stir with a fork until the dough leaves the sides of the bowl and holds together.
4. Lightly dust the board or pastry cloth and a rolling pin with flour and roll the ball into a circle ⅛ inch (0.32 cm) thick.
5. Fold the rolled pastry in half or roll it around the rolling pin, and place it in a **7-inch** (18-cm) (small) pie plate. Gently unfold or unroll, ease crust into pie plate, and crimp edge. Prick shell.
6. Place pie shell on middle shelf of oven and bake 10 to 12 minutes until lightly browned.

B. Effect of Different Fillings on Palatability of Bottom Crust

Procedure

1. Prepare pastry. Use assigned shortening and follow the basic pastry recipe, doubling recipe if required for a two-crust pie (small, 7-inch [18-cm]) pie).
2. Prepare assigned fillings (four basic types: fresh fruit, cooked fruit, starch thickened, or custard).
3. Evaluate the four finished products, crust, and filling in the chart that follows.

Apple Filling (Fresh Fruit)

Double the basic pastry recipe.			flour	1 tbsp	15 mL
cooking apples peeled and sliced	2–3		sugar (optional)	2 tbsp	30 mL
cinnamon, nutmeg, or other spices	¼ tsp	1.25 mL			

1. Set oven at 425°F (220°C). Follow the basic pastry recipe directions through step 5.
2. Roll out the top crust. Make small cuts for steam to escape.
3. Fill the bottom crust with apple filling. Sprinkle with spices, flour, and sugar.
4. Moisten the edge of the bottom crust with water. Place the top crust on the apples and press the crusts together to seal.
5. Trim surplus dough and crimp the edge.
6. Place the pie on the lower oven shelf. Bake for 15 minutes.
7. Move the pie to the center or top rack, reduce oven temperature to 375°F (190°C) and bake 30 more minutes.

EVALUATION OF PASTRY

Palatability Characteristics	Lard		Hydrogenated Fat		Butter		Margarine		Oil	
	Room Temp.	Refrig. Temp.	Room Temp.	Refrig. Temp.	Room Temp.	Refrig. Temp.	Room Temp.	Refrig. Temp.	Room Temp.	Refrig. Temp.
Rate using a, b, c, etc.										
1. **External appearance** a. Color uniform b. Pale c. Surface breaks										
2. **Internal tenderness** a. Very tender b. Fairly tender c. Crumbly d. Tough e. Mealy										
3. **Flakiness** a. Thin flakes b. Some flakes c. Thick flakes d. No flakes										
3. **Flavor** a. Pleasing b. Tasteless c. Displeasing										

Conclusions:

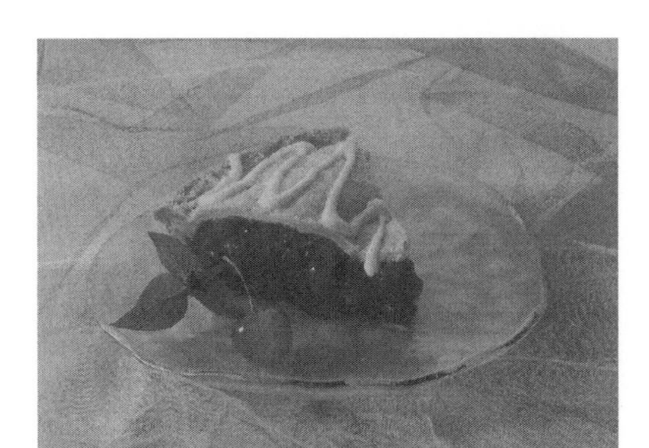

PIE.
Courtesy: SYSCO® Incorporated.

Cherry Pie (Cooked Filling)

Double the basic pastry recipe. Use 1½ cups (360 mL) canned cherry pie filling.

1. Set oven at 425°F (220°C). Follow the directions for basic pastry through step 5.
2. Place the cherry pie filling in the bottom crust, moisten the edge, cover with the top crust, seal, and vent.
3. Place the pie on the lower oven shelf and bake for about 30 minutes, until crust is brown.

Chocolate Meringue Pie (Starch-Thickened)

Follow the basic pastry recipe.

sugar	½ cup	120 mL	egg yolks	2	
flour	3 tbsp	45 mL	vanilla	½ tsp	2.5 mL
milk	1⅓ cups	320 mL	egg whites	2	
square chocolate, chopped	1		sugar	¼ cup	60 mL

1. Set oven at 375°F (190°C). Follow the basic single-crust pastry recipe. Bake 15 minutes.
2. In a saucepan, combine half the sugar and flour. Stir in the milk and chocolate, cooking until the mixture thickens; add the remaining sugar.
3. Slowly add part of the hot mixture to the egg yolks (tempering). Return warmed egg to the chocolate mixture. Cook over low heat, stirring to coagulate the egg.
4. Remove the mixture from the heat; add vanilla. Cool slightly. Pour the filling into the baked pie shell.
5. Set oven at 425°F (220°C). Beat egg whites until soft peaks develop.
6. Add the sugar, about 2 tbsp (30 mL) at a time, beating after each addition.
7. Continue to beat the egg whites until stiff peaks develop.
8. Spread the meringue over the warm, but not hot, filling, spreading to touch the crust.
9. Bake for 4 to 5 minutes or until lightly brown.

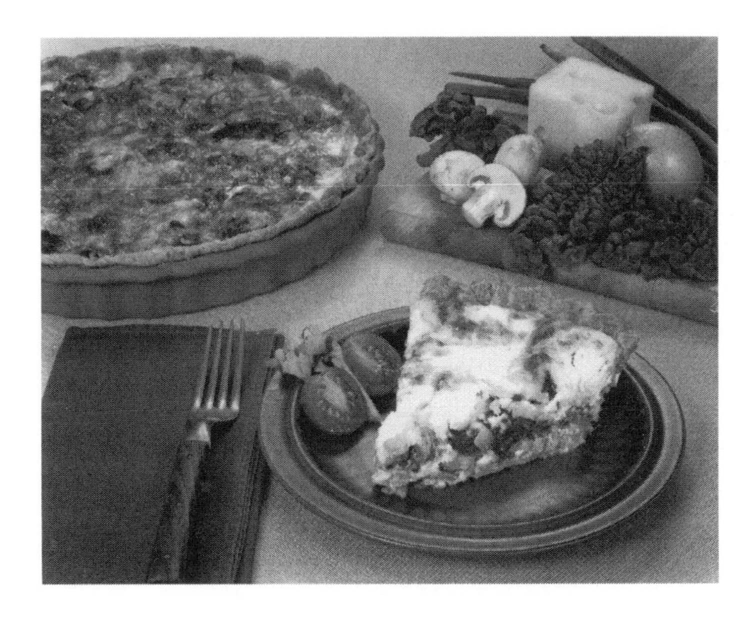

VEGETABLE QUICHE.
Source: Division of Nutritional Sciences, New York State College of Human Ecology at Cornell University, Ithaca, New York.

Quiche (Custard)

Use the basic pastry recipe.[11]

chopped, cooked vegetables[a]	1 cup	240 mL	milk	⅔ cup	160 mL
minced onion	2 tbsp	30 mL	eggs	2	
oregano	¼ tsp	1.25 mL	nutmeg	¼ tsp	1.25 mL
grated cheese	¼ cup	60 mL			

[a] Suitable vegetables include broccoli, asparagus, spinach, or mushrooms.

1. Follow the basic pastry recipe, but bake only 5 minutes. Lower oven temperature to 350°F (175°C).
2. Layer vegetables, herbs, and cheese in crust.
3. Beat milk and eggs and pour over vegetables. Sprinkle with nutmeg.
4. Place pie on lower oven shelf, and bake at 350°F (175°C) 30 minutes. If a knife inserted into the custard does not come out clean, move the pie to the center rack, lower heat to 325°F (165°C), and bake until the custard is firm and the knife comes out clean. Let stand 10 minutes before serving. (Two to three servings)

PALATABILITY OF PIES

Pie	Crust	Filling
Apple		
Cherry		
Quiche		
Chocolate meringue		

[11] Whole wheat or half whole wheat flour suggested.

Delineate the general procedures followed in preparing and baking the crusts for the four basic types of filling used in assigned recipes.

Filling	Procedure with Crust (see recipes)
Fresh fruit	
Cooked fruit	
Starch thickened	
Custard	

QUESTIONS—PASTRY

1. Explain how spreadability of a fat affects texture and tenderness of pastry. Which fat is most spreadable at room temperature? Refrigerated?

2. What is meant by "plastic" when describing a fat? Give an example of a plastic fat.

3. Discuss how hydrogenation changes the characteristics of a fat.

4. What is the cause of a "mealy" textured pastry?

5. In the marketplace, compare the nutrient label panels of several margarines.
   a. What information on the label helps the consumer select a margarine that is high in polyunsaturated fats?

   b. What additives are commonly used in the manufacture of margarines? List several and note the function.

6. a. What difficulty occurs when oil is used in the basic pastry method? Why?

   b. Following is a recipe designed to use oil as the fat in making pastry. Based on your experiences, explain why a tender (not mealy), somewhat flaky pastry can be obtained using this method.

flour, sifted	1 cup	240 mL	oil	¼ cup	60 mL
salt	½ tsp	2.5 mL	milk, cold	2 tbsp	30 mL

   1. Sift flour and salt.
   2. Combine oil and milk, mixing well.
   3. Add liquids all at once to dry ingredients, and stir to form a moist ball.

7. Explain how the following factors affect gluten development in pastry:

Factor	Effect on Gluten	Explanation
Amount of fat		
Plasticity of fat		
Temperature of fat		
Amount of mixing of fat into flour		
Amount of liquid		
Amount of mixing of water into fat-flour		
Mixing ½ whole wheat, and ½ all-purpose flour		

SUMMARY QUESTIONS—BATTERS AND DOUGHS

1. Compare the nutritive value of a similar amount of each of the following grain products:

Grain	Energy (kcal)	Protein (g)	Calcium (mg)	Iron (mg)	Thiamin (mg)	Riboflavin (mg)	Niacin (mg)	Folate (mg)
Wheat flour All-purpose, enriched								
Cake flour								
Whole wheat flour								
Cornmeal Enriched								
Unenriched								
Rye flour								
Soy flour								

2. Complete the following table regarding gluten potential.

Type of Flour	% Protein[a]	Gluten Potential	Uses
Wheat flour Whole wheat	13		
Hard wheat	12		
Soft wheat	9		
All-purpose	10		
Cake	7–8		
Cornmeal	7–9		
Rye flour	34–47		

[a] Source: Watt, B.K. and A.L. Merrill. 1963. ***Composition of Foods.*** Agriculture Handbook, No. 8. Washington, DC: USDA.

3. Analyze the following batters and doughs:

Product	Proportion Liquid/Flour	Ease of Gluten Development	Description of Product with Overdeveloped Gluten
Biscuits			
Muffins			
Pancakes			
Popovers			

4. Indicate how the following variables can affect gluten development in a standard muffin and biscuit recipe:

Ingredient	Muffin	Biscuit
Decreased sugar		
Increased fat		
Increased liquid		
1 cup (240 mL) cornmeal for 1 cup (240 mL) flour		
1 cup (240 mL) bread flour for 1 cup (240 mL) all-purpose flour		

5. What other products besides muffins are prepared by the "muffin" method? What other products are prepared by the "pastry" method?

6. Explain why salt is considered an essential ingredient in yeast breads.

7. What are the functions of a liquid that are common to all batters and doughs?

8. What happens to the following ingredients during baking?

Ingredient	Reaction during Baking
Flour	
Fat	
Milk	
Egg	
Baking powder (double-acting)	

9. List three principal leavening gases, and state the manner in which each may be incorporated into batters and doughs.

10. Could yeast be substituted for baking powder in a biscuit recipe? What changes in procedure would be necessary? Would characteristics of the end product be different? Explain.

11. If biscuits and yeast rolls were each kneaded for 10 minutes, would both products be equally palatable? Explain.

12. Regarding the characteristic of flakiness, describe:
    a. What is meant by flakiness in pastry or biscuits.

    b. How ingredients are manipulated to obtain flakiness.

    c. Why some gluten development is necessary for flakiness.

    d. Why flakiness is not achieved by the muffin method.

13. List several batter and dough convenience foods that are available to consumers.

14. Compare cost and ingredients in three batter and dough convenience foods with those of similar products prepared from "scratch."

15. Potential allergens abound in batter and dough food products. Identify several such food allergens.

Dietitian's Note

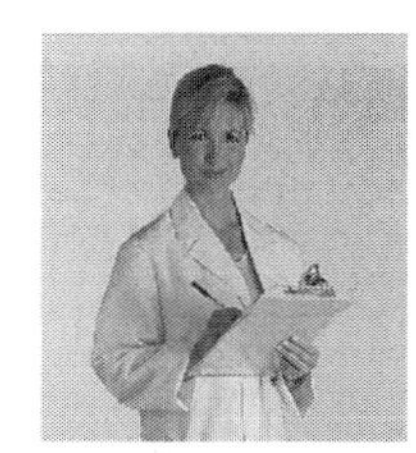

Allergens: Recipes may contain known allergens. See Appendix E.

PART III

Heating Foods by Microwave

Microwave heating and cooking is one way foods are processed and cooked. ***Microwaves***, generated by the magnetron tube of the oven, are waves (such as radio and TV energy ***waves***) absorbed by a food, especially the water, fat, and sugar components. The molecules in the food vibrate at a high rate of speed, billions of times per second, and heat results from this friction. The heat is produced instantaneously in the food and not by delayed transfer from an outside heat source, as occurs with other heat transfer methods. (Think of how one rubs both hands together, to generate heat and warm up on a cold day.)

Microwave cooking is routine for many individuals. It complements conventional cooking methods; however, it does ***not*** replace them for cooking all food, as you know and will see in the lab. This concept and successful uses of the microwave oven may be better understood by preparing the recipes that follow. Microwave cooking may keep the food preparation area cooler, and be quicker and more convenient for our lifestyles. Microwave-ready dinners, entrees, or side dishes are readily available in grocery stores. Major nutrients, as well as important palatability characteristics, are well preserved in microwave cooking, with the exception of vitamin B_{12}.

The microwave oven is more than a "breadbox on the counter." It is more than a way to prepare popcorn or reheat dinners. When one learns how to expand the use of a microwave oven, including use of the probe, memory capacity, and various power-level options correctly, it can be a valuable cooking aid.

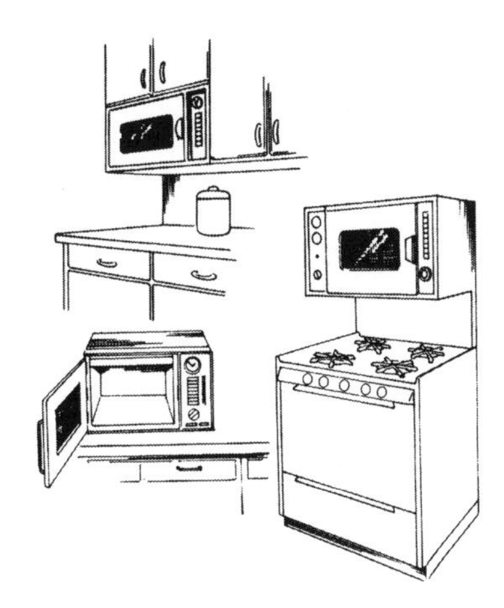

Source: Olson, W. and R. Olson. 1979. North Central Regional Publ. 70-1979. Agricultural Extension Service, University of Minnesota.

Microwave Cooking

When my great-grandfather was a boy,
fast food meant the ones you couldn't catch.

— **Anonymous**

Objectives

To describe how microwave energy heats food
To utilize microwave-cooking procedures for heating a variety of foods
To compare microwave-cooking procedures, utensils, and palatability of final products to conventional cooking
To follow a variety of package instructions for microwaveable products
To delineate the advantages and disadvantages of microwave cooking

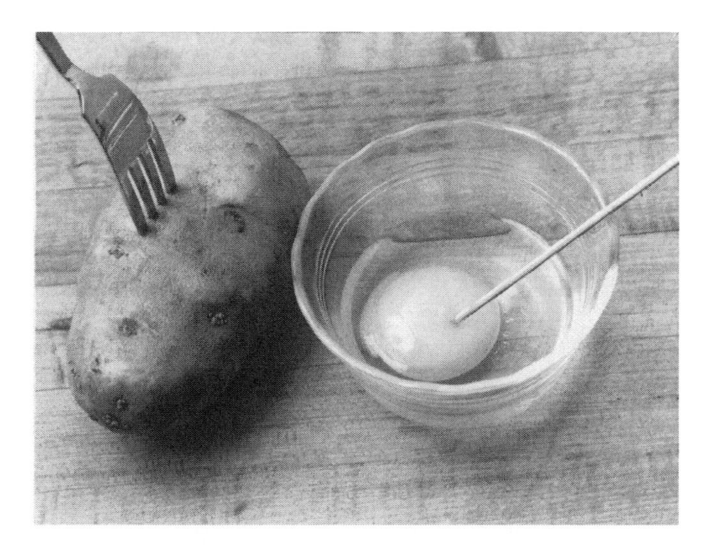

Prick Foods to Release Pressure.
Courtesy: General Electric Company.

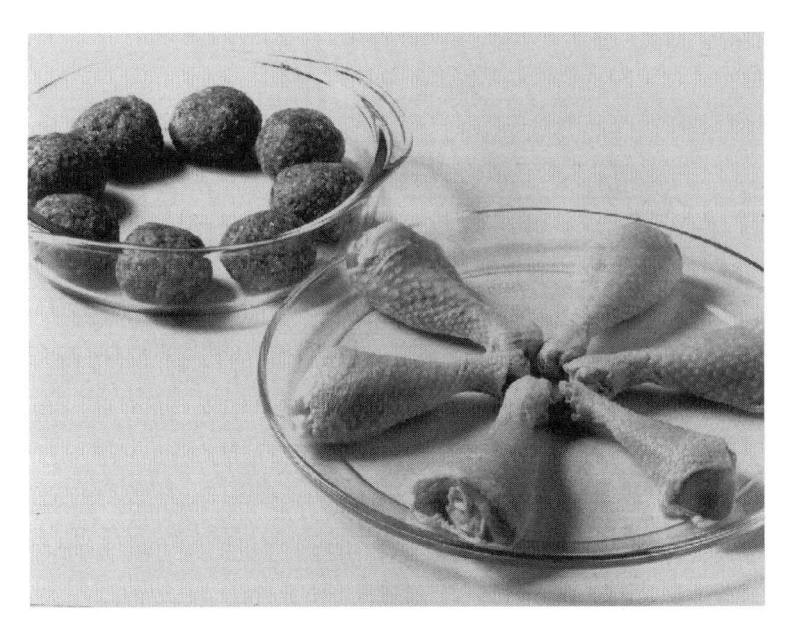

ARRANGE FOODS IN A CIRCLE. IF PORTIONS ARE IRREGULARLY SHAPED OR SIZED, PLACE THICKEST PORTIONS TO THE OUTSIDE OF THE DISH.
Courtesy: General Electric Company.

REFERENCES

Appendices I, L-I, L-II

Watanabe F. et al. 1998. Effects of microwave heating on loss of vitamin B12 in foods. ***Journal of Agricultural and Food Chemistry*** 46: 206–210.

http://ag.arizona.edu/pubs/health/az1081.pdf -Microwave Cooking Basics, Temperatures, Defrosting, Utensils

U.S. Department of Agriculture. 2006 (July). ***Microwave Ovens and Food Safety***. FSIS Fact Sheets. Washington, DC: USDA.

TERMS

- Heat penetration
- Hot spots
- Ionizing/nonionizing
- Magnetron
- Molecular friction
- Shielding
- Thermal runaway

The following exercises using the microwave oven may be completed individually or incorporated into the various exercises of Part II in the manual. Microwave on HIGH setting unless otherwise noted.

> Doubling a microwave recipe may require 1½ the amount of time
> Halving a recipe may require approximately ⅔ the recipe time.

EXERCISE 1: EFFECT OF COOKING PROCEDURE ON PIGMENTS AND FLAVORS

PROCEDURE

1. Prepare 1 cup (240 mL) of assigned vegetables representing pigments and flavor compounds; place in small glass container.
2. Add ¼ cup (60 mL) water and cover tightly with plastic wrap.
3. Microwave for 3 minutes. Remove ½ cup (120 mL) vegetable.
4. Cover tightly and microwave 5 minutes longer.
5. Drain, label, and display both samples. Record observations.

	Cooked 3 Minutes		Cooked 8 Minutes	
Pigments	Color	Texture	Color	Texture
Chlorophyll				
Anthocyanin				
Flavor	Flavor	Texture	Flavor	Texture
Allium				
Brassica				

Conclusions:

EXERCISE 2: FRUITS

PROCEDURE

1. Prepare fruits as directed.
2. Label and display. Record observations.

Applesauce

apples, pared, cored, sliced	2		sugar	1 tbsp	15 mL
water	2 tbsp	30 mL	nutmeg, cinnamon	dash	

1. Place apples and water in small casserole, cover.
2. Microwave 4 minutes, or until tender.
3. Let stand, covered, for 2 minutes. Add sugar and spices; mash, if necessary.

Baked Apples

apples, cored	2	water	2 tbsp	30 mL

1. Slit skin around top center of fruit to prevent bursting during cooking. Place apples in small casserole.
2. Add water, cover, and microwave for 6 minutes or until tender.
3. Let stand, covered, for 2 minutes.

Fruit	Palatability
Applesauce	
Baked apple	

EXERCISE 3: VEGETABLES

General Directions

1. Prepare vegetables by cutting small, uniform pieces, pricking skin, or arranging with more tender parts toward the center of the dish.
2. Add approximately ¼ cup (60 mL) water per pound (454 g) of vegetable.
3. Cover and microwave all vegetables, turning or stirring vegetable halfway through cooking.
4. Evaluate palatability of finished product.

Procedure

1. Follow recipe directions for assigned product.
2. Evaluate palatability and, if possible, compare to like products cooked by conventional methods.

Vegetable	Palatability
Baked potato	
Pennsylvania red cabbage	
Cauliflower	
Baked eggplant with tomato sauce	
Italian vegetable medley	
Baked tomato	
Packaged frozen vegetable; use microwave package instructions	

Baked Potatoes

1. Prick scrubbed potato in two or three places and place on a paper towel in oven.
2. Microwave 5 to 7 minutes, turning potato once or twice during cooking.
3. Let stand, uncovered, 2 minutes before cutting open. Open and top with seasonings.

Pennsylvania Red Cabbage

1. Use ingredients listed in the chapter on Fruits and Vegetables.
2. In a 2-quart (2-L) baking dish combine all ingredients except vinegar.
3. Cover. Cook 6 minutes. Stir and microwave 6 minutes longer. Test cabbage for desired degree of doneness; stir in vinegar. If necessary, microwave longer. Let stand 2 to 3 minutes. (Two to three servings.)

Cauliflower

cauliflower florets	2 cups	480 mL	margarine	1 tsp	5 mL
water	2 tsp	10 mL	dill weed	season	

1. Place cauliflower in 1-qt. (1-L) baking dish.
2. Add water, cover, and cook 6 minutes. Turn dish and continue microwaving 2 to 3 minutes until cauliflower tests done. Let stand 2 to 3 minutes.
3. Add seasonings desired. (Two servings.)

Baked Eggplant with Tomato Sauce

medium eggplant	½		oregano	½ tsp	2.5 mL
tomato sauce	1 cup	240 mL	mozzarella cheese slices	2 1-oz.	57 g

1. Pare eggplant; cut into ⅛-inch (0.3-cm)-thick slices.
2. Spread 2 tbsp (30 mL) sauce on bottom of 1-qt. (1-L) casserole dish.
3. Mix remaining sauce and oregano. Layer eggplant and sauce in casserole dish.
4. Cover and cook 4 minutes. Rotate dish a quarter turn and cook 4 minutes longer. Test to see whether vegetable is tender. If not, cook 2 minutes longer.
5. Place mozzarella cheese on top of eggplant and cook 1 minute longer, until cheese has melted. Let stand 2 to 3 minutes. (Three to four servings.)

Italian Vegetable Medley

broccoli florets	1½ cups	360 mL	sliced carrot rounds	½ cup	120 mL
cauliflower florets	1½ cups	360 mL	green peppers (cut into	2	
fresh mushrooms	4 oz.	114 g	1-inch [2.54-cm] squares)	¼ cup	60 mL
zucchini, sliced thin	1 cup	240 mL	Italian dressing		

1. Arrange vegetables in a 2-qt. (2-L) glass serving dish or pie plate; place broccoli flower side up, around outside, then cauliflower, zucchini, peppers, and mushrooms, and finally carrots in the center.
2. Spoon Italian dressing evenly over all vegetables.
3. Cover and cook 3 minutes or until vegetables are tender. (Six to eight servings.)

Baked Tomatoes

1. Follow the recipe in the chapter on fruits and vegetables for ingredients.
2. In a glass cup, place fat and onion, cover, and cook 1 minute. Mix with bread crumbs and seasonings. Stuff tomatoes.
3. Place stuffed tomato halves in a 1-qt. (1-L) glass casserole dish. Cover.
4. Cook, giving dish a half-turn after half of cooking time. Two halves take 2 to 2½ minutes; 4 halves, 3 to 4 minutes.

EXERCISE 4: STARCH PRODUCTS

Procedure

1. Cook starch items as assigned.
2. Label and display. Record observations.

Starch Product	Palatability
Oatmeal	
Farina	
Basic sauce	
Milk-based variation	
Cinnamon–sugar sauce	
Pudding Butterscotch	
Chocolate	
Other	

A. Pasta, Rice, and Cereals

Pasta and rice take about the same time to cook on the stove and in the microwave oven. Microwave reheating, however, is an excellent way to reheat pasta or rice. To reheat, cover dish tightly with lid, then microwave. (Open lid carefully.)

Oatmeal

oatmeal	⅓ cup	80 mL	water	¾ cup	180 mL

Place ingredients in a 1-qt. (1-L) glass container; cover and cook 3 to 4 minutes.

Cream of Wheat or Farina

cereal	2½ tbsp	37.5 mL	water	1 cup	240 mL

Place ingredients in a 1-qt. (1-L) glass container; cover and cook 3 to 4 minutes.

B. Flour and Cornstarch as Thickeners

Basic Starch-Thickened Sauce

margarine	2 tbsp	30 mL	milk	1 cup	240 mL
flour	2 tbsp	30 mL			

1. Place fat and flour in a 1-qt. (1-lL) casserole. Cook for 2 minutes, stirring after 1 minute.
2. Gradually add milk, stirring.
3. Cook 3½ to 4 minutes, stirring every minute until mixture boils. Yield: 1 cup (240 mL).

Variations for Milk-Based Sauce

Cheese Sauce: To finished sauce add 1 to 2 oz. (28 to 57 g) grated cheddar cheese and a dash of cayenne pepper. Cook 1 minute to melt cheese.

Curry Sauce: Add 1 tsp (5 mL) curry powder with flour and proceed as directed in Basic Sauce.

Cinnamon–Sugar Sauce

sugar	½ cup	120 mL	water	1 cup	240 mL
cornstarch	1½ tbsp	22.5 mL	margarine	1 tsp	5 mL
cinnamon	1 tsp	1.25 mL			

1. Mix half of sugar, cornstarch, cinnamon, and water in a small glass container.
2. Cover and cook 3 to 4 minutes until mixture boils, stirring sauce after 1½ minutes.
3. Add remaining sugar and fat; stir until blended. Yield: 1⅓ cups (320 mL).

Variation
Citrus Sauce: omit cinnamon, add 1 tbsp (15 mL) lemon juice and 1 tsp (5 mL) lemon rind in step 3.

Butterscotch and Chocolate Puddings

Use ingredients listed in the chapter on Cereal and Starch to make puddings. Control addition of ingredients that could adversely affect thickness of starch sol. Follow the directions in the basic starch-thickened sauce recipe (above).

EXERCISE 5: EGGS[1]

CAUTION: Never hard cook eggs or reheat eggs that are in the shell.
Pressure builds up inside and eggs burst.

PROCEDURE

1. Prepare egg products as directed.
2. Label and display. Record observations.

Egg Product	Palatability
Scrambled	
Baked custard	
Fried—browning dish	

[1] Check final temperature of product. DO NOT taste any egg product that does not reach a final cooking temperature of 140°F (60°C), held for 3½ minutes, or 160° (71°C).

Scrambled Eggs

margarine	2 tsp	10 mL	eggs	2
milk	2 tbsp	30 mL		

1. Place margarine in glass bowl or 2-cup (480-mL) measuring cup; microwave on HIGH until melted (about 30 seconds).
2. Add milk, mix. Add eggs, beat with a fork.
3. Cook for 45 seconds on HIGH; stir set portions from outside to center.
4. Cook 45 seconds on MEDIUM; repeat stirring. When finished, eggs should be firm and at 165°F (74°C). Let stand 1 to 2 minutes.

Baked Custard

milk	1 cup	240 mL	sugar	1 tbsp	15 mL
egg	1		vanilla	½ tsp	2.5 mL

1. Beat ingredients until well mixed.
2. Pour mixture into three 6-oz. (180-mL) glass cups.
3. Cook 3 minutes on MEDIUM; rotate oven position and cook for 3 more minutes on MEDIUM. Test for doneness by inserting a clean knife. Continue cooking and testing at 30-second intervals until egg is coagulated. Custard should not boil.

Eggs on Browning Dish

Following manufacturer's directions, fry an egg on a browning dish. Check temperature to ensure safety.

EXERCISE 6: MEAT, POULTRY, AND FISH[2]

PROCEDURE

1. Prepare products as directed.
2. Microwave fish on HIGH, meat and poultry on MED-HIGH for best results.
3. Label and display. Record observations.

Product	Palatability
Baked Fish	
Chicken	
Meatballs	

[2] Review information in Appendices G-I and G-II concerning regulations about cooking temperatures for meat and poultry.

Baked Fish

fish fillet	½ lb	227 g	margarine	2 tsp	10 mL

1. Arrange fish in glass baking dish; dot with margarine.
2. Cover dish with double thickness of wet paper towels.
3. Microwave 4 minutes, rotate dish a half turn, cook 3 more minutes. Test to see if fish flakes. Continue cooking, testing at 1-minute intervals until fish flakes. (Two to three servings.)

Toppings: sweet-sour, tomato, or barbecue sauce.

Chicken

margarine	2 tsp	10 mL	paprika, herbs	season
chicken thighs	2			

1. Place margarine in microwave-safe container; microwave until melted.
2. Place chicken thighs in container, turning to coat with margarine. Arrange meatiest parts toward outside of dish.
3. Sprinkle with seasonings and cover with wax paper.
4. Microwave 5 to 7 minutes on MEDIUM-HIGH. Let stand, covered 5 minutes (1 piece: 3 to 5 minutes; 2½ to 3 lb. [1.14 to 1.36 kg]: 22 to 29 minutes). Chicken is done when clear juice runs from a fork prick.

Meatballs

ground beef	½ lb.	227 g	finely chopped onion	2 tbsp	30 mL
egg	1	60 mL			
bread crumbs	¼ cup				

1. Mix ingredients. Shape into 6 balls.
2. Arrange balls in a circle on a glass pie pan. Cover.
3. Microwave 5 to 8 minutes, rotating dish half-turn after 3 minutes. Microwave 4 minutes, test for doneness. Continue cooking, testing at 30-second intervals until finished. Let stand, covered, 2 to 3 minutes. (Two servings.)

EXERCISE 7: BATTERS AND DOUGH

Procedure

1. Prepare baked products as directed at various power levels.
2. Baked products may be prepared with herbs, spices, or other ingredients in order to provide color.
3. Label and display. Record observations.

Baked Product	Palatability
Muffins	
Biscuits	
Pastry shell	
Other, package instructions	

Muffins

1. Use the ingredients in the basic muffin recipe, in the chapter on Batters and Dough.
2. Once mixed, pour batter into six slightly greased 6-oz. (180-mL) glass custard cups or microwave muffin pan, filling cups half full.
3. Arrange cups in a ring or in a microwave muffin pan.
4. Microwave 3 to 5 minutes on MEDIUM-HIGH. Check for doneness at 2½ minutes. Continue to bake at 30-second intervals until done. Rotate a half-turn at each 30-second interval. Let stand 2 minutes. (Muffins will seem barely set and top may have moist spots, but toothpick inserted in center comes out clean when done.) (Six muffins.)

Biscuits

1. Use the ingredients in the basic biscuit recipe, in the chapter on Batters and Dough.
2. Cut dough into 12 biscuits.
3. Place a drinking glass or glass cup in the center of a greased glass pie plate.
4. Arrange biscuits around the drinking glass, overlapping to fit.
5. Microwave 6 to 8 minutes on MEDIUM, rotating dish a half-turn after 3 minutes. Let stand 2 minutes. (12 biscuits.)

Basic Pastry Shell

flour, sifted	1 cup	240 mL	water	2 tbsp	30 mL
shortening	⅓ cup	80 mL	herbs, spices	to color	

1. Mix ingredients by pastry method. Roll and fit into glass pie plate; prick pastry with fork.
2. Microwave 6 to 7 minutes rotating a half-turn after 3 minutes. Check for doneness: the bottom will be dry and opaque; the top dry, blistered, but not brown.

EXERCISE 8: REHEATING BAKED PRODUCTS

PROCEDURE

1. Place five baked yeast rolls in a circle on a paper towel in the microwave oven.
2. Microwave 10 seconds, and remove one roll. Repeat at 4-second intervals, taking out a roll at each interval.

3. Compare the overall palatability of the reheated rolls.
4. Summarize the results of the experiment.

Roll number	1	2	3	4	5
Time to remove roll	10 seconds	14 seconds	18 seconds	22 seconds	26 seconds
Results					

EXERCISE 9: DEFROSTING

PROCEDURE

1. Place two ¼-lb. (114-g) ground-beef patties on separate plates.
2. Microwave one patty on HIGH for 4 minutes. Microwave the other patty for 4 minutes on DEFROST.
3. Observe the internal quality of the meat. Evaluate the extent of defrosting or cooking that has occurred.
4. Summarize the results below.

Defrosting Method	Quality
High	
Defrost	

SUMMARY QUESTIONS—MICROWAVE COOKING

1. Why do microwave recipes often require that the container be turned during the cooking process?

2. Why is a "rest period" or "standing time" included in directions for microwave recipes?

3. List several ways that the lack of browning in microwave cooking may be overcome.

4. From readings, compare nutrient retention in microwaved vegetables to vegetables cooked by conventional methods. Include any losses that occur in microwaved vegetables.

5. Considering sanitary quality, why do the USDA directions recommend microwaving pork to 170°F (77°C)?

6. Based on experiments, summarize the palatability characteristics of the following microwaved products:

Product	Palatability
Fruits	
Vegetables	
Starches	
Eggs	
Meats, poultry, fish	
Batters, dough	

7. In defrosting foods, why is a low setting rather than a high one used?

8. Do containers used for microwave cooking get hot? Explain.

9. How do directions on packaged microwaveable food products assist the consumer? Note any suggestions for improvements in package directions.

10. State some recipe changes that must be made in converting from cooking with a conventional oven to cooking with a microwave oven.

11. Are all foods successfully prepared in the microwave oven? Specify what quality standards are not met using microwave cooking.

PART IV

Meal Management

Now comes mealtime! Meals should be personally satisfying and obtainable within our resources, such as time, money, knowledge, and energy. In consideration of the multifaceted dimensions of food, we view how economics, individual taste, lifestyle, cultural and ethnic background, and special nutritional needs affect meal planning for individual and group mealtime.

The suggested meal management project options provided here give you an opportunity to apply creatively the principles of food selection as well as safe, nutritious, and fun food preparation. Go for it!

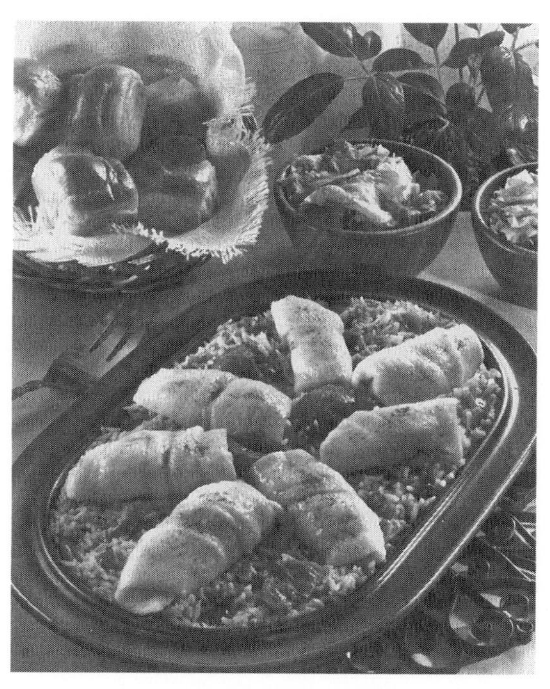

Courtesy: R.T. French Co.

Meal Management

A smiling face is half the meal.

— Latin proverb

He who eats alone chokes alone.

— Arab proverb

Objectives

To apply principles of nutrition, sanitary quality, economics, and the science of food to meal planning
To adapt meal plans to a variety of cultures, including international and regional domestic menu patterns
To adapt meal plans to low cost, low calorie, and other modifications
To demonstrate basic food preparation skills, use of equipment, time management, and service of food
To identify food product allergens and acceptable recipe alternatives
To identify strategies for eating out

References

Appendices E, L

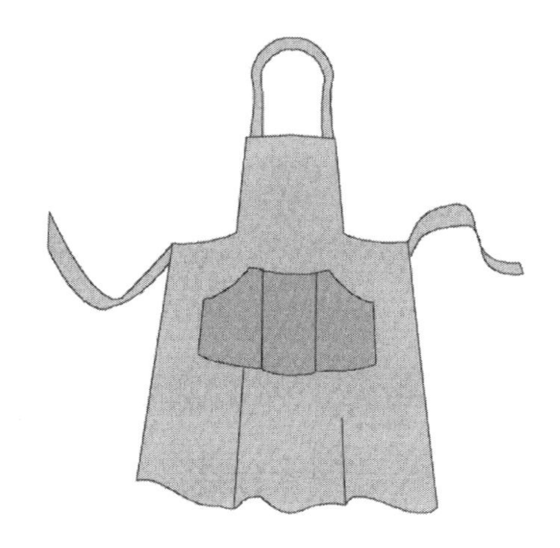

Terms

Appendices K, L-1, L-2

EXERCISE 1: ANALYZING MENUS FOR PALATABILITY QUALITIES

PROCEDURE

Using the following chart of menus, identify planning errors and then make suggestions for improvements in the palatability of the meals, for example, color, texture, and so forth. Where relevant, also note how nutritional aspects could be improved.

Menu	Planning Errors	Improvements
Salmon Red beans and rice Lima beans Lettuce salad Tiramisu Tea		
BBQ pork on a bun French fries Buttered carrots Broccoli spears with cheese sauce Baked rice pudding Milk		
Curried eggs on rice Lettuce wedge, vinaigrette dressing Roll and butter Gingerbread Nonfat milk		
Ham-lentil soup, crackers Grilled cream cheese sandwich Waldorf salad Apple turnover with cheese Milk		
Cream of chicken soup, crackers Cottage cheese and sliced peach salad Baked custard Milk		

EXERCISE 2: ECONOMIC CONSIDERATIONS IN MENU PLANNING

PROCEDURE

Adapt the following high-cost foods to moderate- and low-income budgets, if possible.

High-Cost Food	Moderate-Cost Food	Low-Cost Food
Calves' liver		
Ground sirloin		
Fresh orange juice		
Frozen halibut		
Fresh salmon		
Center slice ham		
Porterhouse steak		
Packaged baked sweet rolls		
Fresh tomatoes		
Whole milk, fluid		
Aged sharp cheddar cheese		
Fresh asparagus tips		
Leaf lettuce		
Butter		
Frosted cornflakes		
Frozen chocolate cream pie		
Packaged hash brown potatoes		
Frozen pancakes		

EXERCISE 3: LOW-CALORIE MODIFICATIONS

PROCEDURE

The following menu[1] totals approximately 2600 to 2700 calories. Adapt this plan for an individual who wishes to consume 1600 to 1700 calories.

Food	Portion	Modifications
Breakfast		
Orange juice (fresh)	¾ cup (180 mL)	
Scrambled egg	1 large	
Bacon	1 slice	
Bagel with	1	
Cream cheese	2 tbsp (30 mL)	
Jam	1 tsp (5 mL)	
Milk, whole	1 cup (240 mL)	
Water, tea, or coffee		
Brown bag lunch		
Ham sandwich, sliced ham	3 oz. (85 g)	
Lettuce	2 leaves	
Mayonnaise	1 tbsp (15 mL)	
Whole wheat bread	4 slices	
Bean salad	1 cup (240 mL)	
French dressing	2 tsp (10 mL)	
Chocolate chip cookie	1	
Apple	1 medium	
Blueberry yogurt	1 cup (240 mL)	
Water, tea, or coffee		
Dinner		
Vegetable chowder, milk base	1 cup (240 mL)	
Baked fish with tomato sauce	5 oz. (140 g)	
Buttered broccoli spears	½ cup (120 mL)	
Mixed green salad: lettuce, spinach, green onions, cucumbers	1½ cup (360 mL)	
Blue cheese dressing	2 tbsp (30 mL)	
Gingerbread	1 serving	
Pear (fresh)	1 medium	

[1] Adapted from U.S. Department of Agriculture. 1981. Ideas for Better Eating. Washington, DC: USDA.

EXERCISE 4: MEAL PLANNING

The class will divide into groups, with each group producing a meal with the same meal-planning guidelines found in the chart below. Include salad/appetizer, main dish, starch, vegetable(s), garnish/ accent, dessert, and beverage.

SUGGESTIONS FOR MEAL PLANNING (CATEGORIES)		
Low-calorie	Regional United States	Vegetarian
Low-cholesterol	International meals	Preschool, nursing home, camp
Low-sodium	Oven meals	Eating with allergies (unspecified allergy)
Low-fat: 30% kcal	Stovetop meals	
Low-income	Crock-pot cooking	

PROCEDURE FOR THE MEAL PREPARATION

1. Prior to the Meal Day:
   a. Plan. Within the framework of one of the suggested meal plans, plan a full day's menu (only the lunch or dinner will be prepared in the laboratory), with consideration for palatability—for example, food preferences, color, texture, shapes, flavor, and temperature of foods—as well as cost.

   b. Submit:
      i. Market Order. Worksheet A.
      ii. Nutritive value of the meal selected, including calories, fat, protein, carbohydrate, cholesterol, sodium, calcium, iron, vitamin A, and vitamin C. The percent of calories from carbohydrate, protein, and fat may be calculated. (A computer-generated analysis may be used in lieu of the one appearing here.)
      iii. Recipes for the one meal you are preparing.
      iv. Cost per day per person, the cost per lunch or dinner per person. (Follow any specifications if given.)
      v. Planning Schedule. Worksheet B page. The meal should be prepared in _______ hours.

2. On the Meal Day: Prepare Meal (Exercise 5).

3. After the Meal:
   a. Submit Analysis of Criteria Used (Worksheet C).
   b. Submit Exercise 5, Student Evaluation.

Worksheet A

Market and Equipment Order

Materials Needed	Amount Needed	Cost
Cereal products		
Produce		
Frozen products		
Canned products		

Meats/eggs		
Fats/oils		
Sugars/sweeteners		
Miscellaneous		
Equipment/materials needed		

WORKSHEET B

PLANNING SCHEDULE

Date of Meal Preparation: Name:

Meal Prepared: (attach)

1. Work out a time schedule for the preparation of your meal.

Time	Preparation Steps

2. Diagram complete table setting (cover), noting placement of food on plates and serving dishes, serving utensils, and centerpiece.

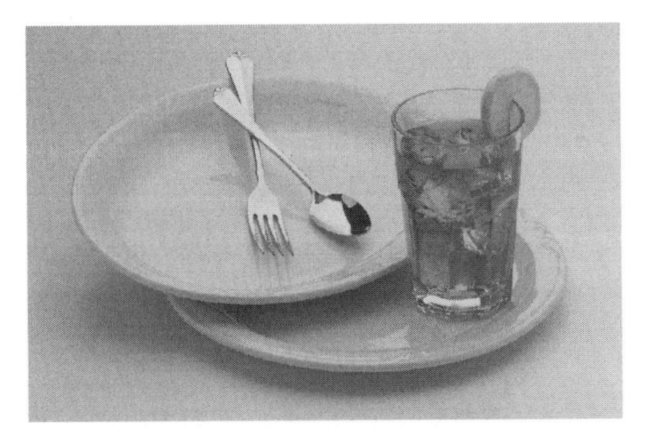

Courtesy: SYSCO® Incorporated.

Worksheet C

Summary Analysis of Meal Plan

Evaluate your completed meal plan, noting the criteria you established and the various strategies you used to meet the criteria (nutrition, good sanitation, etc.). Where appropriate include specific examples.

Criteria	Strategies

Use additional pages if necessary for a complete analysis.

EXERCISE 5: MEAL PREPARATION

PROCEDURE

1. Prepare approved meal with assigned classmate(s) to meet allocated time schedule.
2. Serve meal.
3. Evaluate the completed meal, noting specific examples of strategies employed to achieve a successful meal.
4. Instructor will evaluate the following:
    - Adherence to time schedule
    - Food science principles
    - Cooking techniques
    - Palatability of meal
    - Table setting and ease of service
    - Kitchen organization and cleanup
    - Use of equipment
    - Completeness of self-evaluation

STUDENT EVALUATION OF THE PREPARED MEAL

Menu for the day (student will attach)

1. Complete Budget of Time and Money:

Factor	Budgeted	Expended	Comments
Time			
Money			

2. Evaluate palatability:

Characteristic	Good	Fair	Poor	Suggestions for Improvement
Color				
Texture				
Shape or form				
Temperature				
Satiety				
Flavor				
Degree of doneness				

3. List sanitary precautions taken during the preparation and service of the meal.

4. Select one cooked product prepared for the meal and analyze the recipe for the application of food science principles:

Product Name:

Step	Principles

EXERCISE 6: RESTAURANT MEALS—FOOD-ORDERING PRACTICES

PROCEDURE

1. Survey several classmates regarding their food-ordering practices.
2. Complete the following chart and place a checkmark according to food-ordering practices. (The restaurants chosen may include any type of restaurant.)

Food-Ordering Practices	Sometimes	Always	Never	Comments (such as type of restaurant)
Ordering based on economics				
Ordering based on nutrition				
Order à la carte				
Order table d'hôte (grouped-price meals)				
Order dessert				
Method of ordering: Dining in at a restaurant				
Drive-through				
Phone order				
Other (specify)				
Order dessert				
Order other (specify)				

Conclusions:

SUMMARY QUESTIONS—MEAL MANAGEMENT

1. Why are the aesthetics of menu planning and service important?

2. In planning, which nutrients must be planned in specific amounts?

3. The recommended dietary allowance (RDA) for iron is frequently difficult to meet. How can the absorption of iron be enhanced? What dietary factors inhibit iron absorption?

4. Identify advantages and disadvantages of using established food guides (e.g., the Food Pyramid, *Dietary Guidelines*) for meal planning.

5. In planning meals for low-income levels, which foods or food groups could be increased (because of their excellent nutritive value for dollars spent)? Which could be decreased?

6. Identify factors, other than cost, that may make planning low-income meals difficult.

7. Provide examples of how the inclusion of restaurant foods in the diet may affect an individual's food choices in menu planning.

8. What are some of the physical limitations that make preparing and/or eating common foods difficult for some individuals?

9. What are the nutritional concerns of a person with food allergies, a vegetarian, and a person who never has enough time to eat breakfast (attach)?

10. Attach a checklist to evaluate sanitation practices to be used when you prepare food. Consider food buying, storage, and preparation of meal preparation.

11. Identify advantages of menus offering customers two ways of purchasing—à la carte, table d'hôte.

12. Indicate on the thermometer the temperature or range of temperatures for the following:
    a. Lukewarm, scalding, simmering, poaching

    b. Gelatinization of wheat/corn starch

    c. Coagulation of whole egg

    d. End boiling temperature of sugar syrup for crystalline product

    e. End boiling temperature of sugar syrup for amorphous product

    f. Oven temperature for baking: soufflé in water bath; soufflé without water bath; biscuits; popovers; pastry

    g. Internal temperature for rare, medium, and well-done meat

    h. Temperature for holding of foods

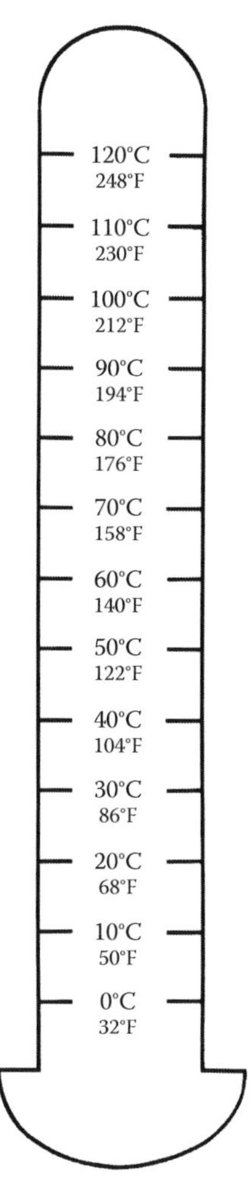

Source: Division of Nutritional Sciences, New York State College of Human Ecology at Cornell, Ithaca, New York.

Appendices

The following Appendices A through P are referenced in chapters throughout this manual. To remain current and most informed, it is recommended that additional material be reviewed.

Appendix A
Legislation Governing the Food Supply[1]

Laws Enforced by the Food and Drug Administration

The Food and Drug Administration (FDA) is a federal regulatory agency responsible for enforcing laws to protect consumers of foods, drugs, cosmetics, medical devices, chemical products, and other articles used in the home. Congress enacts the laws and relies on the FDA to establish necessary regulations and standards, and, thereafter to enforce the regulations and standards (FDA).

The Federal Food, Drug, and Cosmetic Act—1938

The Food, Drug, and Cosmetic Act replaced the original Food and Drug Act of 1906 with new and stronger provisions. The following regulations of this law refer to foods:

- Food must be pure and wholesome, safe to eat, and produced under sanitary conditions. Adulterations and misbranding are defined.
- Labeling must be truthful and informative
- Provisions are stated for establishing standards of identity, quality, and fill.

Standards of Identity prevent adulteration by defining exactly what a specific food must contain. For example, fruit jams must contain at least 45 parts of fruit and 55 parts of sugar or other sweetener.

Standards of Quality set minimum specifications for such factors as tenderness, color, and freedom from defects in canned fruits and vegetables. For example, quality standards for canned foods limit the "string" in green beans, excessive peel in tomatoes, hardness in peas, and "soupiness" in cream-style corn.

Standards of Quality should not be confused with Grades A, B, C, Prime, Choice, Fancy, and so forth, which are set by the U.S. Department of Agriculture (USDA). Manufacturers pay USDA for this voluntary service.

Standards of Fill tell the packer how full the container must be to avoid deception of the consumer and charges of "slack filling."

---

[1] Choose websites used throughout this manual to obtain current information!

The law provides for enforcement through inspection, collection of samples, and prosecution in the courts.

Miller Pesticide Amendment—1954

This amendment sets safety limits for pesticide residues allowed on raw agricultural commodities.

Poultry Products Inspection Act—1957

This act regulates poultry and poultry products, including labeling.

Food Additive Amendment—1958

Key points of this amendment are:

- Prohibits the use of new additives until manufacturer has established its safety.
- Establishes a list of additives, generally recognized as safe (GRAS). This list was drawn up after a review of available evidence showed no significant risk from the intended use of the additive.

  Since 1970, the FDA has been reassessing the safety of additives on the GRAS list. A panel of scientists, established under an FDA contract with the Federation of American Societies for Experimental Biology (FASEB), has reviewed all experimental evidence to determine if continued use of additives on the GRAS list is justified. Consumers can expect the safety assessment of additives to continue and perhaps the GRAS list will be revised in light of additional scientific data.
- Contains a statement known as the Delaney Clause. This clause states that no food additive can be approved by the FDA for human food if it is found to induce cancer when ingested by humans or animals. The Delaney Clause does not recognize any level of cancer-producing chemical as safe.

Color Additives Amendment—1960

This amendment allows the FDA to establish by regulation the condition for safe use of color additives in food.

Fair Packaging and Labeling Act—1966

This act requires that consumer products in interstate commerce be honestly and informatively labeled. The FDA is empowered to enforce provisions that affect foods, drugs, cosmetics, and medical devices. The Federal Trade Commission (FTC) administers the law with regard to other products.

Because there are existing federal laws governing the labeling of meat products, poultry, and poultry products, these foods are excluded from the provisions of the Fair Packaging and Labeling Act and are monitored by the USDA.

Some specific points of this act in regard to food labels are:

- The label must state the name and address of the manufacturer, packer, or distributor of the food.
- The label must show the common or usual name of the product.
- The ingredients must be listed on the label in descending order of their predominance by weight in the product. Exceptions are some foods for which standards of identity have been established. The ingredient descriptions of standardized foods are on file with the FDA.

- Additives used in food products must be listed on labels. This ruling also applies to standardized foods, with the exception of butter, cheese, and ice cream.
- A statement of the net weight or volume of contents must appear on the main display label of the package.
- Weights between 1 pound and 4 pounds net weight must also be stated in total number of ounces, so cost per ounce can be figured easily.
- Labels must not carry misleading terms that qualify units of measure such as "giant quart" or "jumbo pound."
- The FDA has authority to limit the amount of packaging material or air space to the amount that is required to protect the contents of the package, or which is required by the kind of machinery used to package the commodity.

Food Labeling Regulations—1973

Label regulations were established by the FDA to provide the consumer with valuable tools for identifying and selecting nutritious foods. The components of the program were interrelated and called for several new concepts in food labeling, such as identifying and giving amounts of nutrients in a food product, establishing nutritional quality guidelines for certain foods, or giving the percentage of the characteristic component in a product.

The regulation specified methods and formats of labeling products intended ***for special dietary needs.*** It established a standard of identity for ***dietary supplements,*** including vitamins, minerals, and highly enriched foods. This regulation required use of "imitation" when a food was nutritionally inferior to a food product for which it is a substitute. Foods containing any amount of artificial flavor were to be labeled with the name of the food and characterizing flavor preceded by the words "artificial" or "artificially flavored."

Nutrition Labeling and Education Act (NLEA)—1990

As a result of the NLEA there are regulations that specify information food processors must include on their labels, such as Nutrition Facts. There is extensive, mandatory nutrition labeling of food, standard serving sizes, and use of health claims. The purpose of the NLEA is to:

- Assist consumers in selecting foods that can lead to a healthier diet.
- Eliminate consumer confusion.
- Encourage production innovation by the food industry.

The FDA set 139 reference serving sizes for use on Nutrition Facts labels that more closely approximates amounts consumers actually eat than previous labeling. General descriptive terms allowed for use on food labels were provided.

1992: The FDA's voluntary point-of-purchase nutrition information for raw produce and fish.

1994: The Food Safety and Inspection Service (FSIS) of the USDA introduced regulation for voluntary nutrition labeling of raw meat and poultry. May 8, 1994 was the deadline for meeting NLEA requirements for labeling with "Nutrition Facts" panel on packaging.

Pathogen Reduction: Hazard Analysis and Critical Control Point (HACCP) System Regulation—1996

This regulation codifies principles for the prevention and reduction of pathogens and requires the development of Sanitation Standard Operating Procedures (SSOPs) and a written HACCP plan that is monitored and verified by inspectors of meat and poultry processing plants.

The FDA Modernization Act of 1997

The FDA Modernization Act of 1997 (FDAMA) was passed by the Senate and the House, and signed into law in 1998. It amends the FD&C Act, and the biological products provisions of the Public Health Service Act (PHS Act), with the intent "… to improve the regulation of food, drugs, devices, and biological products, and for other purposes." The Act ***eliminates*** the FDA's ***mandatory premarket approval*** for use of the majority of substances that come into contact with food, or may migrate into it. Instead, manufacturers must provide 120 days of notification to the FDA. Among other sections that address drugs, devices, and biological products, the FDAMA contains nine *food* petitions as separate sections of the ruling.

- Flexibility for Regulations Regarding Claims—Section 301
- Petitions for Claims—Section 302
- Health Claims for Food Products (authoritative statements, yet not FDA)—Section 303
- Nutrient Content Claims (significant information, 120 days)—Section 304
- Referral Statements (such as "see side panel for nutrition information")—Section 305
- Disclosure of Irradiation (size of statement, and use of symbol)— Section 306
- Irradiation Petition (to control food contamination with pathogens)—Section 307
- Glass and Ceramic Ware (regarding FDA's ban on ceramics)—Section 308
- Food Contact Substances (including the safety of additives)—Section 309

Allergen-Free Labeling (see Appendix E)

The Food Allergen Labeling and Consumer Protection Act of 2004 (FALCPA) requires that food manufacturers identify foods that contain the presence of ***protein*** derived from crustacean shellfish, eggs, fish, milk, peanuts, soybeans, tree nuts, or wheat. It is known that food allergies may present on the skin, in the respiratory tract, or perhaps in the intestines. Allergy testing concurrent with normal eating (no dietary restriction at or prior to testing) may reveal specific food allergens. Of course, each human body may be its own diagnostic laboratory when it comes to dietary sensitivity.

General Labeling

Complete information about food must be supplied on food packages. It must include the following:

- Name of product, name, and place of business
- Net weight—ounces (oz.), or pounds and ounces
- Ingredients—listed ***by weight in descending order*** on ***ingredients list*** (not Nutrition Facts portion) of label

- Company name and address
- Product date if applicable to product
- Open date labeling—voluntary types able to be read by the consumer
  - Expiration date—deadline for recommended eating (i.e., yeast)
  - "Best if used by" date—date for optimum quality, QA, or freshness
  - Pack date—date food was packaged
  - Pull date—last day sold as fresh (i.e., milk, ice cream, deli)
- Code date—read only by manufacturer
- Nutrition information—"Nutrition Facts" on nearly all labels
- Nutrient content claims substantiated
- Health claims used only as allowed
  - Other information
  - Religious symbols—such as Kosher (if applicable)
  - Safe handling instructions—such as on meats
  - Special warning labels—alcohol, aspartame that may affect select consumers
  - Product code (UPC)—bar code

Health Claims: Some Examples of Approved Model Health Claims Used on Food Labels

- Calcium and lower risk of osteoporosis (if along with regular exercise and a healthy diet)
- Sodium and a greater risk of hypertension (high blood pressure)
- Saturated fat and cholesterol and a greater risk of coronary heart disease
- Dietary fat and a greater risk of cancer
- Fiber-containing grain products, fruits, and vegetables and a reduced risk of cancer
- Fruits, vegetables, and grain products that contain fiber (particularly soluble fiber) and a reduced risk of heart disease
- Fruits and vegetables and a reduced risk of cancer
- Folate and neural tube defect
- Sugar alcohols and reduced risk of tooth decay
- Soluble fiber from certain foods and risk of coronary heart disease (CHD)
- Soy protein and risk of CHD
- Whole grains and reduced risk of heart disease and certain cancers
- Plant sterol and plant stanol esters and reduced risk of CHD
- Diets high in potassium and low in sodium and reduced risk of high blood pressure and stroke

For more food laws and regulations, see:

http://www.ift.org/divisions/food_law/ IFT Food Laws and Regulation Division

http://www.iflr.msu.edu/ Institute for Food Laws and Regulations

http://www.lib.berkeley.edu/doemoff/govinfo/federal/gov_legfood.html Food Policy Legislation

http://www.fda.gov/SiteIndex/default.htm

http://www.fda.gov/Food/FoodSafety/HazardAnalysisCriticalControlPointsHACCP/default.htm milk, seafood

Pending legislation:

1. HR875 Food Safety Modernization Act of 2009:
    - Introduced and referred to committee, to establish the Food Safety Administration within the Department of Health and Human Services to protect the public health by preventing food-borne illness, ensuring the safety of food, improving research on contaminants leading to food-borne illness, and improving security of food from intentional contamination, and for other purposes.
    - This is a bill in the U.S. Congress originating in the House of Representatives ("H.R."). A bill must be passed by both the House and Senate and then be signed by the president before it becomes law.
2. Summary of Discussion Draft of the Food Safety Enhancement Act of 2009. General Provisions:
    1. *Creates an up-to-date registry of importers.* Requires all importers of drugs, devices, and foods to register with the FDA annually and to pay a registration fee.
    2. *Requires unique identification numbers for facilities and importers.* To enhance information about FDA-regulated entities, creates unique identification numbers for all drug, device, and food facilities and importers.
    3. *Creates a dedicated foreign inspectorate.* Requires FDA to establish and maintain a corps of inspectors to monitor foreign facilities producing food, drugs, devices, and cosmetics for American consumers.
    4. *Grants FDA new authority to subpoena records related to possible violations.*
    5. *Provides protection for whistleblowers who bring attention to important safety information.* Prohibits entities regulated by the FDA from discriminating against an employee in retaliation for assisting in any investigation regarding any conduct which the employee reasonably believes constitutes a violation of federal law.

Appendix B
Food Guides and Dietary Guidelines

FOOD GUIDES

Food grouping systems are designed to provide a simple, organized method of helping people plan an adequate and balanced diet. The most widely used system today is the Food Pyramid introduced in 2005 by the U.S. Department of Agriculture (USDA). In this guide, foods are classified into one of five groups depending on the similarity of their nutritive value. Each group (for 12 classifications of age and gender, etc.) provides some but not all of the nutrients needed to maintain good health, and no one group is more important than another. The Food Pyramid lists the groups and the recommended number of servings from each group. Serving sizes within each group provide approximately similar amounts of the major nutrients. The Fats, Oils, and Sweets are *not* a major food group.

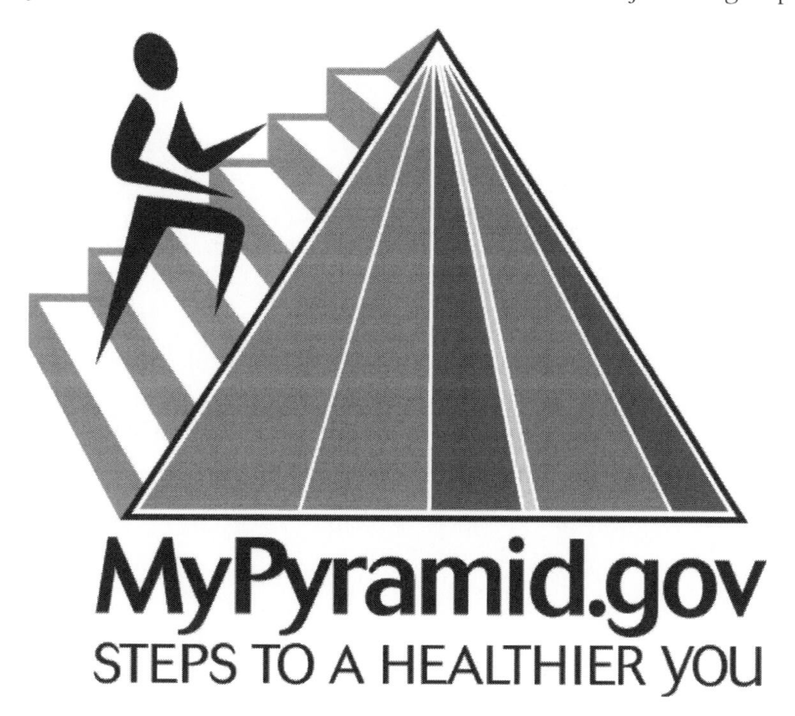

USDA MyPyramid.
Source: U.S. Department of Agriculture.

www.mypyramid.gov:

- Education Framework: http://www.mypyramid.gov/downloads/MyPyramid_education_framework.pdf
- Getting Started: http://www.mypyramid.gov/downloads/MyPyramid_Getting_Started.pdf
- Anatomy of MyPyramid: http://www.mypyramid.gov/downloads/MyPyramid_Anatomy.pdf
- Sample Menu at 2000 calories: http://www.mypyramid.gov/downloads/sample_menu.pdf

Because most foods can readily be placed in one of the food groups, the Food Pyramid easily adapts to usual eating patterns, as well as various cultural and ethnic food choices. For example, tortillas and grits would be classified under the Breads Group and papayas and mango under Fruit. Some mixed foods, for example, macaroni and cheese, need to be broken down to their component parts for placement in food groups; macaroni would be placed in the Breads Group and cheese in the Milk Group.

Additional multicultural food guides are available from Penn State Nutritional Center.

Dietary Guidelines

http://www.health.gov/dietaryguidelines/dga2005/chronology.htm
http://www.healthierus.gov/dietaryguidelines
http://www.nhlbi.nih.gov/health/public/heart/hbp/dash/

The **Dietary Guidelines for Americans**, 2005, gives science-based advice on food and physical activity choices for health. See the full 80-page Dietary Guidelines report.

http://www.health.gov/dietaryguidelines/dga2005/document/

Many Americans are concerned that their diets are too high in energy, fat, sugar, and sodium, and too low in fiber. These dietary imbalances have been associated with high incidence of chronic diseases such as heart disease and cancer. In response to this concern, the USDA and the Department of Health and Human Services developed the *Dietary Guidelines for Americans*. The guidelines are designed for healthy people over 2 years old.

These guidelines stress good eating habits based on variety and moderation. In contrast to the Food Pyramid that suggests food choices to obtain an adequate supply of all nutrients, the *Guidelines* were developed to help moderate dietary excesses. Used together, the Food Pyramid and *Dietary Guidelines* are simple and effective tools to help the selection of a well-balanced diet without excess. See MyPyramid.gov—Portion sizes of foods (see IB).

What Is a "Healthy Diet"?

The Dietary Guidelines describe a **healthy diet** as one that

- Emphasizes fruits, vegetables, whole grains, and fat-free or low-fat milk/milk products;
- Includes lean meats, poultry, fish, beans, eggs, and nuts; and
- Is low in saturated fats, *trans* fats, cholesterol, salt (sodium), and added sugars.

Of course, all of these foods do not fit into special diets followed by persons with allergies (Appendix E). The recommendations in the ***Dietary Guidelines*** and in MyPyramid are for the general public over 2 years of age. MyPyramid is not a therapeutic diet for any specific health condition. Individuals with a chronic health condition should consult with a health care provider to determine what dietary pattern is appropriate for them.

See MyPyramid.gov—Portion sizes of foods (see IB).

Appendix C
Some Food Equivalents

Protein Equivalents[a] (16–20 g)		
milk	2¼ cups	540 mL
cottage cheese	½ cup	120 mL
cheddar-type cheese	2½ oz.	70 g
meat	3 oz	85 g
eggs	3	
cooked dried beans/peas	1 cup	240 mL
peanut butter	5 tbsp	75 g
hot dogs	2½	
walnuts, almonds, cashews	¾ cup	180 mL
bread slices	8	
prepared dry cereal	8 oz.	227 g
cooked macaroni	3 cups	720 mL
cooked rice	4 cups	950 mL

Calcium Equivalents[b] (270–320 mg)		
whole milk	1 cup	240 mL
nonfat milk	1 cup	240 mL
buttermilk	1 cup	240 mL
yogurt	1 cup	240 mL
ice cream	1½ cups	360 mL
cheddar cheese	1⅓ oz.	37 g
creamed cottage cheese	1¼ cup	300 mL
cream cheese	1 lb.	454 g
oranges	6	
ground beef	6 lb.	2.72 kg
bread slices, enriched	14	
cooked broccoli, kale	2 cups	480 mL
cooked collard greens	1 cup	240 mL

Vitamin C Equivalents (60–70 mg)		
orange	1	
orange juice	½ cup	120 mL
grapefruit	¾ cup	180 mL
cantaloupe	½	
strawberries, whole	¾ cup	180 mL
watermelon	1/16	
green pepper	¾	
tomato	1½	
tomato juice	1½ cups	360 mL
kale, turnip greens, cooked	1 cup	240 mL
collards, cooked	¾ cup	180 mL
broccoli, cooked	½ cup	120 mL
spinach, cabbage, cooked	1¾ cups	300 mL
potatoes, white or sweet	3	

Iron Equivalents[c] (4–5 mg)		
whole grain enriched bread	8 slices	
cooked dried beans/peas	1 cup	240 mL
ground beef	4 oz.	114 g
liver	1½ oz.	43 g
clams, canned	4 oz.	114 g
eggs	4	
plums, canned	2 cups	480 mL
prune juice	½ cup	120mL
dried apricots	½ cup	120 mL
tomato juice	2 cups	480 mL
peas, canned	1 cup	240 mL
peas, cooked	1½ cups	360 mL
spinach, cooked	1 cup	240 mL
white potatoes, medium	5	

[a] Protein equivalent refers to ***amount*** of protein, not quality of protein.

[b] Spinach and rhubarb have substantial amounts of calcium, but it is complexed with oxalate and not fully utilized.

[c] Availability of iron in eggs and plant sources may be less than indicated.

Appendix D
Average Serving or Portion of Foods[a,b]

Item	Weight/Amount		Item	Weight/Amount	
A. Dairy Products			**F. Fruits**		
Cheese			Fresh	By the piece	
Cheddar	1–2 oz.	28–57 g	Fresh, cut up: canned	½ cup	120 mL
Cottage	¼–½ cup	60–120 mL	Fruit juices	½ cup	120 mL
Milk			**G. Meat**		
For drinking	1 cup	240 mL	Fresh, frozen, canned, cooked	2–3 oz.	57–85 g
For cooked cereal	2 oz.	60 mL	Liver	2 oz.	57 g
For dry cereal	4 oz.	120 mL	Bacon	2 slices	
Ice cream	½ cup	120 mL	Frankfurters	2	
Yogurt	½–1 cup	120–240 mL	Lunch meat	2 slices	
B. Eggs			**H. Plant Protein**		
Fried, poached, hard/soft	1		Legumes, beans, cooked	1½ cups	360 mL
Scrambled	1½		Peanut butter	2–4 tbsp	30–60 mL
C. Fats and Oils			Nuts, seeds	¼ cup	60 mL
Butter or margarine	2 tsp	10 mL	**I. Poultry, cooked**		
Salad dressing	2 tbsp	30 mL	Chicken, turkey, boned	3 oz.	85 g
Mayonnaise	1 tbsp	15 mL	Chicken, broiler	½ bird	
D. Fish, Shellfish			Chicken, fryer	¼ bird	
Cooked	2–3 oz.	57–85 g	**J. Vegetables**		
E. Bread and Cereals			Cooked, canned	½ cup	120 mL
Bread, rolls, muffins	1		Lettuce	¼ head	
Cereals, cooked	½–¾ cup	120–180 mL	Asparagus	3–6 spears	
Cereals, dry	¾–1 cup	28 g	Brussels sprouts	4–6	
Macaroni, rice, cooked	½ cup	120 mL	Corn, ears	1	
Saltines	4		Potatoes, whole (medium)	1	

[a] These may not be amounts personally consumed. Knowledge of the average quantity per serving is useful in estimating cost and nutritive value.

[b] See FDA standard serving sizes on food labels for individual foods.

Recommended Servings for Different Energy Intakes

Food Group	1600 kcal	2200 kcal	2800 kcal
Bread	6	9	11
Vegetable	3	4	5
Fruit	2	3	4
Milk	2–3	2–3	2–3
Meat	2–3 (5 oz.)	2 (6 oz.)	2–3 (7 oz.)

Source: Adapted from USDA. Recommended servings.

Standard Serving Size Finder

Food	Serving Size	Example
Bread		
Bread	1 slice	audio cassette
Cornbread	1 piece	bar of soap
Pancake	1	CD
Pasta	1 cup	fist
Rice	½ cup	scoop size
Ready-to-eat cereal	1 oz.	½–1¼ cups
Vegetables		
Chopped vegetables	½ cup	light bulb
Raw leafy vegetables	1 cup	baseball size
Baked potato	1 medium	fist
Raw carrot sticks	7–8	
Fruit		
Fresh fruit	1 medium	tennis ball; fist
Cut fruit	½ cup	fist
Raisins and dried fruit	¼ cup	large egg
Dairy		
Milk	1 cup	
Cheese	1½ oz.	9-volt battery
Ice cream	1 cup	baseball
Meat, poultry, seafood	3 oz.	deck of cards
Baked fish	3 oz.	checkbook
Dried beans	½ cup cooked	light bulb
Nuts	cup	woman's handful
Peanut butter	2 tbsp	ping-pong ball
Fats		
Margarine/butter	1 tsp	1 pat
Salad dressing	2 tbsp	ping-pong ball

Source: Adapted from USDA.

Appendix E
Food Allergies

The intent of this appendix is to play a small role in introducing the topic of food allergies. Various food allergies may exist either known or unknown in the population. A person's MD or a board-certified allergist should conduct a patient diagnosis; a registered dietitian may advise on food consumption.

These eight foods (typically their protein) account for 90% of food allergens.

- Milk
- Eggs
- Fish
- Crustacean shellfish
- Peanuts (a PEA and not a NUT)
- Soybeans
- Tree nuts (almonds, cashews, and so forth)
- Wheat

Avoiding the above foods can be a challenge, and be careful, because these foods may be ingredients in a wide array of commercially prepared foods and household recipes!

Scientific evidence may also implicate additional foods for some individuals.

THE FOOD ALLERGEN LABELING AND CONSUMER PROTECTION ACT OF 2004 (FALCPA)

This act requires that food manufacturers identify allergenic foods. Allergen food labeling is required after or adjacent to the ingredients list if a food may or does contain allergens.

The most common food allergy symptoms include:

- Tingling in the mouth
- Hives, itching, or eczema
- Swelling of the lips, face, tongue, throat, or other parts of the body
- Wheezing, nasal congestion, or trouble breathing
- Abdominal pain, diarrhea, nausea, or vomiting
- Dizziness, lightheadedness, or fainting

Anaphylaxis
In some people, a food allergy can trigger a severe allergic reaction called anaphylaxis. This can cause life-threatening symptoms, including:

- Constriction and tightening of airways
- A swollen throat or a lump in your throat that makes it difficult to breathe
- Shock, with a severe drop in blood pressure
- Rapid pulse
- Dizziness, lightheadedness, or loss of consciousness (Mayo Clinic)

THE FOOD ALLERGY INITIATIVE (FAI), THE FOOD ALLERGY AND ANAPHYLAXIS NETWORK (FAAN), AND THE CENTER FOR SCIENCE IN THE PUBLIC INTEREST (CSPI)

It has been suggested that perhaps labels should just say "wheat" or say "milk products" in order to be clear regarding ingredient food allergens. In manufacturing, production processes may need to be isolated (dedicated lines or operations) to assure food integrity.

Scientists estimate that approximately 12 million Americans suffer from food allergies (FAAN). Regarding children and allergies, the Centers for Disease Control and Prevention (CDC) states that children may "outgrow" their allergies (http://www.cdc.gov/nchs/data/databriefs/db10.htm). A CDC 2008 report cites 3 million children with food or digestive allergies (http://www.cdc.gov/media/pressrel/2008/081022.htm). This is an 18 percent increase in allergies over the previous 10-year period. Some implicating factors for this increase may be attributed to hygiene, food processing, and global food availability issues. Other factors include less food diversity and more environmental toxins that may get into our food and water supply. As well, children eat more than they did 10 years ago.

ALLERGIES, INTOLERANCES

In addition to food ***allergies***, some persons may experience food ***intolerance***. That intolerance may not be to a protein either. For example, ***lactose intolerance*** involves:

> "lact–*ose*"—a milk sugar. A food ***allergy*** signifies the production of antibodies in response to ingestion of an allergen. Food ***intolerances*** do not produce antibodies. Signs of adverse reactions to food include stomachaches, headaches, rapid pulse rate, nausea, wheezing, hives, bronchial irritation, coughs, and other such discomforts. (Whitney and Rolfes 2008)

Avoidance or elimination of foods causing adverse reactions is the correct course of action.

For more information on food intolerance, see the website http://www.webmd.com/digestive-disorders/celiac-disease/features/gluten-intolerance-against-grain.

Allergen-Free Labeling—Read Labels!

An issue that relates to *food safety* is the manufacture of allergen-free foods. As one *Food Engineering* author has said, "Food safety is being redefined to include allergen-free as well as pathogen-free" (Higgins 2003).

The FDA is responsible for ingredient labeling, and has given notice to food processors that exemptions from ingredient labeling are not tolerated. A food product must contain what it states on the label, and it should ***not*** contain an ingredient it does ***not*** disclose. Life-threatening allergens must be reported on the food label, and in uncertain cases, statements such as "may contain" are displayed as a safeguard.

See the website http://www.fns.usda.gov/fdd/facts/nutrition/foodallergenfactsheet.pdf for more information.

By law, if an allergen is detected following product distribution, ***product recalls*** may be necessary. Recalls are after the fact and can be troublesome. They may be costly in terms of dollars, well-being, and reputation. Either an independent lab or allergen test kits may authenticate that products are allergen-free. Testing is part of industry's good manufacturing practices (GMPs).

According to the director of the Office of Scientific Analysis and Support at FDA's Center for Food Safety and Applied Nutrition "both FDA and food companies are looking harder for allergens ... allergic consumers are becoming more aware of the allergens in foods, and ... [there are] improved allergen-detection methods" (FDA website, http://www.fda.gov/Food/FoodSafety/FoodAllergens/default.htm).

Other Labeling—Gluten-Free

One in 133 people shows sensitivity to gluten (Mahan and Escott-Stump 2008). Gluten is the protein from wheat, oats (unless processed on dedicated production lines), rye, and barley. Specifically, in the case of celiac disease, gluten may flatten the villi in the small intestine, resulting in malabsorption or death. "Unlike some childhood food allergies, which are sometimes outgrown, celiac disease stays with you throughout your lifetime. The most common age at diagnosis now is about 40, and most patients have had at least 10 years of symptoms before diagnosis" (International Food Information Council [IFIC]). Also, eating ***gluten-free*** is not limited to persons diagnosed with celiac disease.

SYMPTOMS OF CELIAC DISEASE

- Malabsorption—vitamins and minerals
- Chronic fatigue and weakness
- Abdominal pain, bloating, gas
- Indigestion/reflux ("heartburn")
- Nausea and vomiting
- Diarrhea, constipation, or both intermittently
- Lactose intolerance
- Weight loss (CD also in obese)
- Bone/joint pain
- Easy bruising of the skin

(continued on next page)

SYMPTOMS OF CELIAC DISEASE

(continued)

- Easy bruising of the skin
- Edema of hands and feet
- Migraine headaches
- Depression
- Mouth ulcers (canker sores)
- Menstrual irregularities
- Infertility (both women and men)
- Recurrent miscarriages
- Elevated liver enzymes
- Dermatitis herpetiformis (DH) is another form of celiac disease.

Source: Case, S. 2006. ***Gluten-Free Diet: A Comprehensive Resource Guide***. Case Nutrition Consulting, Regina, Saskatchewan, Canada. www.glutenfreediet.ca.

In addition to celiac disease, there also exists gluten ***intolerance***, without antibody production. The lifelong remedy is to omit gluten from the diet (Case 2006).

Allergy testing concurrent with normal eating (no dietary restriction at or prior to testing) may reveal specific food allergens. Of course, each human body may be its own diagnostic laboratory when it comes to dietary sensitivity.

"Gluten-Free" is not a labeling requirement; however, often it is apparent on diverse food labels, assisting many persons in their food selection. There exists a plethora of gluten-free baked goods, including apple pie, bagels, breads, brownies, cakes, cookies, and crackers. Some vinegars and soy sauce are specified as "gluten-free" because others may be derived using wheat. As well, there are gluten-free restaurants! "Since food and beverage manufacturers are continually making improvements, food-allergenic persons should read the food label for every product purchased, each time it is purchased" (International Food Information Council).

The following articles on food allergies may be of interest.

PROTEIN BEHIND FOOD ALLERGIES IDENTIFIED

Researchers led by M. Cecilia Berin at Mount Sinai School of Medicine, New York, showed for the first time that CD23, a protein normally present in a person's intestinal tract, acts as a receptor for IgE, a protein associated with allergic reactions.

The researchers studied nine paediatric patients aged three to 17 years. They believe that the presence of CD23 may provide a surrogate method of looking at the gut without invasive tests like biopsies, reported the science portal ***EurekAlert***.

Food allergies are an exaggerated immune responses in which the body produces histamines and antibodies that induce symptoms in the gastrointestinal tract, airways and skin, and in the most severe cases induces anaphylactic shock, an often fatal systemic reaction.

Food allergies often present a unique problem for allergy testing since not every patient has detectable levels of immunoglobulin E (IgE) in their serum, especially patients with delayed allergies.

Source: http://www.bio-medicine.org/medicine-news/Protein-Behind-Food-Allergies-Identified-12497-1/.

FOOD, FOOD ALLERGIES AND MULTIPLE SCLEROSIS

The relationship between food and MS is paradoxical. Though not a cause, food fuels the disease and the development of increasingly disabling symptoms. Yet on the other hand, a careful diet can lead a person back to full recovery from this chronic, degenerative disease. Please note that all the foods implicated as allergens are the same food groups identified as problematic in other diseases.

WHAT IS MS?

Multiple sclerosis is a degenerative disease of the central nervous system in which damage to the protective myelin sheaths and the nerves result in a myriad of symptoms. The loss of nerve conduction can manifest in any body system or organ producing mild or totally debilitating symptoms. There is no full understanding of this disease. However, it is known that in one disease pathway a series of cascading events fuels the disease once it has manifested. The activated immune cells cross the blood brain barrier into the central nervous system where they subsequently attack the myelin and nerves. The other, primary disease pathway is neurodegenerative, though the mechanism is not known. From the good results obtained by the diet, dietary changes are effective with this as well.

THE MS RECOVERY DIET

The main tenets of the diet approach are first to stop the disease process by not eating those foods that activate the immune cells, thereby stopping the cascade of events that lead to symptoms. The second is to eat those foods that assist the body in repair and recovery, thus returning full function. Simply put, once the disease has manifested, there are foods that harm and foods that heal.

The diet recommends greatly reduced intake of saturated fats to less than 15 grams a day and reduced intake of sugar of all forms. Both sugar and saturated fat act on the blood brain barrier. Five groups of foods are most often found to be the allergens that activate the immune cells in the blood stream: wheat and gluten-containing grains, dairy, eggs, yeast and legumes. As a person progresses in recovery they will often find some unique food allergens or triggers.

Equally important to recovery are foods that heal. These include lean protein, especially fish with its essential fatty acids. At least 4 to 10 teaspoons of the essential fatty acids in the healthy oils should be ingested daily (omega 3 fish and flax seed oils, omega 6 vegetable oils). Eat plenty of vegetables and some fruits as well as nongluten grains. The emphasis is on foods rich in antioxidants, raw foods for enzymes and probiotics.

Drink water, get plenty of sunshine (vitamin D), and exercise. Reclaim your life-movement, mind and energy.

Source: Ann D. Sawyer, MSW, LCSW

Some of the best industry practices for allergen control relate to the following (Vaclavik and Christian 2008):

- R&D/product development
- Engineering and system design with dedicated production lines
- Vendor certification of raw materials and ingredients
- Production scheduling to include longer production runs
- Rework segregated
- Labeling and packaging with the right product going into the right package, and ingredients listing to match the actual food product!
- Sanitation—A HACCP-like approach
- Training

Sometimes the consumer is ***unaware*** of the fact that he or she has food allergies, and checks off "no known allergies" (nka) on the patient medical form at the physician's office. On the other hand, perhaps when dining out together, most family members or friends ***know*** that they have allergies or intolerances, thus the wait staff may expect a plethora of questions before a menu item is selected! Diligence in food selection may be necessary for good health.

In summary, there are eight common food allergens. These food allergens, as well as food intolerances, may present with a variety of symptoms, not limited to a skin rash or respiratory distress. Both currently, and looking to the future of food production, there may be increased food allergy concerns. For example, some seeds, tree nuts, and legumes are ingredients increasingly added to a variety of foods, and their small quantities may not warrant food labeling that informs customers.

As Hippocrates stated: "Let food be your medicine, and medicine be your food"!

REFERENCES

Case, S. 2006. *Gluten-Free Diet. A Comprehensive Resource Guide.* Regina, Saskatchewan, Canada: Case Nutrition Consulting. www.glutenfreediet.ca.

Higgins, Kevin T. 2003. A practical approach to allergen control. *Food Engineering*, March 29. http://www.foodengineeringmag.com/Articles/Feat**ure_Article/5bea68ea032f8010VgnVCM100000f.

International Food Information Council/IFIC, Washington, D.C.

Mahan, L.K. and S. Escott-Stump. 2008. *Krause's Food and Nutrition Therapy*, 12th edition. St. Louis, MO: Saunders Elsevier.

Sawyer, A.D. and J.E. Bachrach. 2007. *The MS Recovery Diet.* New York: Penguin Books. www.msrecoverydiet.com.

The Food Allergen Labeling and Consumer Protection Act of 2004 (FALCPA). http://www.cfsan.fda.gov/~dms/alrgact.html.

Vaclavik, V.A. and E.W. Christian. 2008. *Essentials of Food Science*, 3rd ed. New York: Springer.

Whitney, E. and S.R. Rolfes. 2008. *Understanding Nutrition*, 11th ed. Belmont, CA: Wadsworth.

Further information regarding food allergies may be found with the FDA, USDA, CDC, ADA, IFT, and other sites. (Note: Websites listed here are subject to changes/updates of their content.)

Additional references may be found by searching under the following:

Food allergies
"challenge diet"—htp://www.webmd.com/allergies/allergies-elimination-diet
"rotation diet".

Appendix F
Food Additives

An additive is "a substance or a mixture of substances, other than a basic foodstuff, which is present in a food as a result of an aspect of production, processing, storage or packaging" (National Research Council Food Protection Committee).

Every food additive used in processing should serve one or more of the following purposes:

- Improve or maintain nutritional value
- Enhance quality
- Reduce wastage
- Enhance consumer acceptability
- Improve keeping quality
- Make the food more readily available
- Facilitate preparation of the food

In its broadest sense, a food additive is any substance added to food. By legal definition it is any substance the intended use of which results or may reasonably be expected to result—directly or indirectly—in its becoming a component or otherwise affecting the characteristics of any food." *Exempt* categories from the food additive regulation process are GRAS and prior-sanctioned substances.

Many people think of any additive added to foods as a complex chemical compound, although salt, baking soda, and vanilla are commonly used in foods today. The common *lay usage* of the term "food additive" differs from the *legal definition*.

FUNCTIONS OF FOOD ADDITIVES

Basic functions of some food additives are described below. For each classification, examples of additives and their uses in specific foods are provided.

Antioxidants—Antioxidants combine with available oxygen and are added to halt oxidation reactions, to prevent rancidity in fats, oils, cereals, crackers, potato chips, and other foods, and to extend shelf life. They prevent or inhibit oxidation of unsaturated fats and oils, colors, and flavorings. Ascorbic acid and the tocopherols are naturally occurring antioxidants. Synthetic antioxidants include butylated hydroxyanisole (BHA), butylated hydroxytoluene (BHT), tertiarybutylhydroxyquinone (TBHQ), and propyl gallate. Nitrites function as antioxidants to fix the color, flavor, and stability of cured meat.

Bleaching and Maturing Agents—Freshly milled flour has a yellowish color and relatively poor baking quality. If stored for several months, the flour "ages," that is, whitens in color and improves in baking quality. Because natural aging is slow and costly and insect or rodent infestation is difficult to control during storage, chemicals are added to speed the process. Benzoyl peroxide exerts only a bleaching action. The oxides of nitrogen, chlorine dioxide, nitrosyl chloride, and chlorine both bleach and mature flour.

Bulking Agents—Bulking agents such as sorbitol, glycerol, and polydextrose (glucose, sorbitol, and citric acid in 89:10:1 ratio) are used in small amounts to provide body, smoothness, and creaminess, which supplement the viscosity and thickening properties of hydrocolloids.

Coloring Agents—Food colors are used to make processed food look more appetizing by imparting a characteristic color. Baked goods, candy, dairy products (e.g., butter, margarine, and ice cream), gelatin desserts, and jams and jellies often contain color additives. Natural food colors used include annato extract (yellow), cranberries, beet juice, tomatoes (red), carotene, saffron (yellow-orange), and turmeric.

Curing Agents—Curing agents impart color and flavor to foods such as bacon, frankfurters, ham, and salami. They also have antimicrobial properties, which lower the temperature needed to kill ***Clostridium botulinum***. They inhibit the growth of ***Clostridium perfringens, Staphylococcus aureus,*** and nonpathogens.

Edible Films and Waxes—Edible films such as the polysaccharides cellulose, pectin, starch, and vegetable gums, or proteins such as casein and gelatin may be applied with a thin coat to foods. Edible waxes are applied to fruits and vegetables to improve or maintain appearance, prevent mold, and contain moisture, while still allowing respiration. Food-grade ***vegetable waxes,*** including petroleum-, beeswax-, and shellac-based wax or resin, and food-grade ***animal-based*** waxes are regulated as GRAS.

Emulsifiers—Emulsifiers are surface-active agents and have the ability to surround small droplets of fat, thereby dispersing them throughout a mixture. Emulsifiers are used in cake mixes, confections, ice cream, salad dressings, and shortenings to improve uniformity of performance. Some common emulsifiers are mono- and diglycerides, lecithin, and polysorbates. The presence of emulsifiers affects the texture of starch products and they are sometimes included to improve the texture of dehydrated potatoes and to help retain the softness of bread.

Enzymes—Enzymes are nontoxic substances that occur naturally in foods, catalyzing various reactions. They are easily inactivated by pH and temperature. Bromelain (from pineapple), ficin (from figs), and papain (from papaya) are used as meat tenderizers. Amylases hydrolyze starch in flour, invertase is used to hydrolyze sucrose in candy, pectinases clarify pectin-containing jellies or juices, and proteases are used in cheese making and soy sauce production.

Fat Replacers—Fat replacers include carbohydrate-, fat-, and protein-based substances such as maltodextrins, sucrose polyesters of fatty acids and sucrose, and microparticulated protein, respectively.

Firming Agents—Firming agents such as calcium chloride improve processed fruits or vegetables by hardening or firming the texture.

Flavoring Agents—Flavoring agents, both natural and synthetic, make up the largest group of food additives and are used in baked products, confections, ice cream, prepared meats, and soft drinks. Natural flavoring substances include herbs, spices (e.g., salt, pepper, cloves, ginger) and sweeteners, essential plant oils (citrus), and extractives (vanilla extract). Synthetic flavors include amyl acetate (banana), benzaldehyde (almond, cherry), citral (lemon), and flavor enhancers such as monosodium glutamate (MSG).

Humectants—Humectants or moisturizing agents prevent such foods as coconut and candy from drying. Examples include polyhydric alcohols such as glycerol, propylene glycol, mannitol, and sorbitol that are used to improve texture and retain moisture because of their affinity for water.

Nutrient Supplements—Historically the term ***enrichment*** has denoted the process of adding vitamins and minerals to processed foods to compensate for losses incurred during processing, storage, and distribution. ***Fortification*** has referred to the addition of a nutrient deemed lacking in the diet to an appropriate food. "Except for foods with specific standards, the two terms often are used interchangeably in food labels."[1] The FDA defines both terms as the addition of nutrients to food.[2] Thiamin, riboflavin, niacin, iron, and folate,[3] and in some instances, calcium and vitamin D are added to milled grains. The FDA has established standards of maximum and minimum amounts of these nutrients for enrichment of corn grits, cornmeal, farina, macaroni, noodle products, rice, and wheat flour. Vitamins A and D may be added to margarine; vitamin D to both fluid and evaporated milk; vitamins A and D to fluid and nonfat dry milk. In many regions of the United States, iodine is added to table salt.

pH Control Substances—Natural or synthetic acid or alkali ingredients change or maintain the initial pH of a product. For example, the tart taste of soft drinks and fruit drinks is achieved through the use of organic acids, natural or synthetic. Acids, alkalis, buffers, or neutralizing agents may also be used as flavor additives or to preserve food. For example, acid ingredients lower the pH of foods and inhibit microbial growth. Acetic acid, citric acid, organic acids from apples or figs (malic acid), lactic acid, or tartaric acid may be useful as additives, the latter for leavening. Calcium propionate is added to control the pH of breads.

Preservatives—Food additives may be used to delay natural deterioration, not to disguise it. Food can deteriorate through microbial growth of molds, bacteria, and yeast, and through reaction with oxygen, which may alter flavor, color, and texture. Inhibitors such as vinegar, salt, and sugar are used in pickles, sauerkraut, jams, and jellies. The vinegar is acidic, and the salt and sugar compete with bacteria for water and therefore lower the water activity (A_w). Other additives with these functions, calcium or sodium propionates and potassium sorbate, are additives used to control mold in bread and bacilli growth, which causes "rope" in breads or mold. Sodium benzoate inhibits yeast and mold in confections, fruit juices, margarine, and pickles. A preservative may be used alone or in combination with other additives or preservation techniques such as cold or heat preservation, or dehydration.

Sequestrants—Sequestrants such as EDTA (ethylenediaminetetracetic acid) and pyrophosphate form inactive complexes with metallic ions that can catalyze fat oxidation or the formation of cloudy precipitates. Additionally, they prevent metals from catalyzing reactions of pigment discoloration, flavor or odor loss, or vitamin oxidation. Sequestrants are added to carbonated beverages, cooked hams, margarine, salad dressings, canned shrimp and tuna, and vinegar.

Stabilizers and Thickeners—Stabilizers and thickeners are used to give a smooth, uniform texture to many foods. The presence of stabilizers and thickeners prevents the separation of chocolate particles in chocolate milk, keeps ice crystals smaller in ice cream, imparts "body" to artificially sweetened beverages, and maintains uniform texture in puddings and confections. Included in this group of additives

[1] Thonney, P. and C. Bisogni. 1983. ***Fortified and Enriched Foods. You Should Know about Food Ingredients***, 6, No. 2. Division of Nutritional Sciences, Cornell University, Ithaca, NY.

[2] ***Federal Register***, January 25, 1980.

[3] ***Federal Register***, March 5, 1996.

are alginates (from kelp), carrageenan (a seaweed derivative), dextrins of starch and modified starches; hydrocolloids (material that holds water) such as gelatin (e.g., the protein from animal bones, hoofs), vegetable gums such as gum tragacanth, gum arabic, guar, and locust bean, and pectin; and cellulose compounds such as methylcellulose, carboxymethylcellulose (CMC), and sorbitol.

Other miscellaneous food additives include *anticaking agents, dough conditioners, fumigants, leavening agents, lubricants, propellants,* and *artificial* and *natural sweeteners.*

Appendix G
pH of Some Common Foods

pH	Food	pH	Food
2.0	Limes	5.2	Turnips, cabbage, squash
2.1		5.3	Parsnips, beets
2.2	Lemons	5.4	Sweet potatoes, bread
2.3		5.5	Spinach
2.4		5.6	Asparagus, cauliflower
2.5		5.7	
2.6		5.8	Meat, ripened
2.7		5.9	
2.8		6.0	Tuna
2.9	Vinegar, plums	6.1	Potatoes
3.0	Gooseberries	6.2	Peas
3.1	Prunes, apples, grapefruit (3.0–3.3)	6.3	Corn, oysters, dates
3.2	Rhubarb, dill pickles	6.4	Egg yolk
3.3	Apricots, blackberries	6.5	
3.4	Strawberries, lowest acidity for jelly	6.6	Milk (6.5–6.7)
3.5	Peaches	6.7	
3.6	Raspberries, sauerkraut	6.8	
3.7	Blueberries, oranges (3.1–4.1)	6.9	Shrimp
3.8	Sweet cherries	7.0	Meat, unripened
3.9	Pears	7.1	
4.0	Acid fondant, acidophilus milk	7.2	
4.1	Commercial mayonnaise (3.0–4.1)	7.3	
4.2	Tomatoes (4.0–4.6)	7.4	
4.3		7.5	
4.4	Lowest acidity for processing at 100°C	7.6	
		7.7	
4.5	Buttermilk	7.8	
4.6	Bananas, egg albumin, figs, isoelectric	7.9	
4.7	Point for casein, pimientos	8.0	Egg white (7.0–9.0)
4.8		8.1	
4.9		8.2	
5.0	Pumpkins, carrots	8.3	
5.1	Cucumbers		

Source: Reprinted by permission from ***Handbook of Food Preparation,*** 6th ed. American Home Economics Association, Washington, DC. 1975.

Appendix H-1
Major Bacterial Foodborne Illnesses[1]

	Salmonellosis (Infection)	*Staphylococcus* (Intoxication)	*Perfringens* (Infection/Intoxication)	Botulism (Intoxication)
Causes	*Salmonella* (facultative) Bacteria widespread in nature, live and grow in intestinal tracts of human beings and animals.	*Staphylococcus aureus* (facultative) Bacteria fairly resistant to heat; bacterial toxin produced in food is extremely resistant to heat. Toxin produces illness.	*Clostridium perfringens* (anaerobic) Spore former. Vegetative cells destroyed with thorough cooking; spores can survive to germinate, and numbers grow.	*Clostridium botulinum* (anaerobic) Spore-forming organisms that grow and produce a potent neurotoxin.
Symptoms	Severe headache, followed by vomiting, diarrhea, abdominal cramps, and fever. Infants, elderly, and persons with low resistance most susceptible. May cause death in these groups.	Vomiting, diarrhea, prostration, abdominal cramps.	Nausea without vomiting, diarrhea, acute inflammation of stomach and intestines.	Dizziness, double vision, inability to swallow, speech difficulty, progressive respiratory paralysis. Fatality rate is high unless diagnosed promptly and an antitoxin given.
Onset	6–72 hours	1–6 hours	8–22 hours	12–36 hours
Duration	2–3 days	24–48 hours	24 hours or less	Fatal if untreated.
Source	Transmitted by eating contaminated food, or by contact with infected persons or carriers of the infection. Also transmitted by insects, rodents, and pets; domestic and wild animals.	Transferred to foods by humans from hands, nasal passages, infection, and skin abrasions.	*Note:* Caused by large numbers of this bacteria (infection) in a food which, after ingested, produces a toxin in the gut (intoxication).	Toxin in food.
Foods	Eggs; poultry, red meats, unpasteurized dairy products	Custards; eggs; meat, and meat products; warmed-over foods	Large cuts of meats, stews, soups, or gravies that have been kept on steam tables for long periods of time or cooled slowly.	Canned low-acid foods; smoked fish; stews; honey for infants; baked potatoes in foil; large quantities of sautéed vegetables kept unrefrigerated overnight.
Prevention	Avoid cross-contamination. Cook all meats thoroughly, and cook poultry and eggs to 165°F (74°C). Cool quickly.	Proper heating and refrigeration. Good personal hygiene. Toxin is destroyed only by boiling several hours or in a pressure cooker for 30 minutes at 240°F (115.5°C).	Time-temperature control in cooling and reheating meat. Maintain foods out of the temperatures between 45°F (7°C) and 140°F (60°C).	Bacterial spores destroyed by high temperatures obtained only in a pressure canner. (More than 6 hours at boiling point needed to kill spores.) Toxins destroyed with 10–20 minutes of boiling, depending on food density. Keep sous-vide packages refrigerated.

[1] Cross-contamination spreads bacteria to other foods. Sanitize hands, work surfaces, and utensils.

Appendix H-1 (cont'd)
Major Bacterial Foodborne Illnesses

	Listeriosis (Infection)	*Bacillus cereus* (Intoxication)	Campylobacteriosis (Infection)	*Escherichia coli* 0157:H7 (Infection/Intoxication)
Causes	*Listeria monocytogenes* (facultative); can grow in damp environment	*Bacillus cereus* (facultative)	*Campylobacter jejuni*	*Escherichia coli* 0157:H7
Symptoms	Meningitis in immuno-compromised individuals. Nausea, vomiting, headache, fever, chills.	Nausea, vomiting, diarrhea, abdominal cramps.	Diarrhea, fever, headache, nausea, abdominal pain.	Bloody diarrhea, diarrhea, nausea, severe abdominal pain, vomiting, occasionally fever.
Onset	1 day to 3 weeks	8–16 hours (can be ½–5 hours)	3–5 days	12–72 hours
Duration	Indefinite. High fatality in immunocompromised individuals.	Less than 12 hours	1–4 days	1–3 days
Source	Humans; also domestic wild animals, soil, water, mud.	Soil and dust.	Domestic and wild animals.	Humans (intestinal tract), cattle, and other animals.
Foods	Unpasteurized milk and some soft cheese products; raw meat/poultry; chilled, ready-to-eat foods; raw vegetables.	Cooked rice and rice dishes, and cereal products; food mixtures; spices; sauces; vegetable dishes; meatloaf. Especially a problem where large batches of foods are prepared ahead and improperly cooked/reheated.	Unpasteurized milk and dairy products; untreated water; raw vegetables; undercooked meats.	Raw and undercooked red meats, unpasteurized milk, and fruit juices, cream-baked pies.
Prevention	Use only pasteurized milk and dairy products. Cook foods to proper temperature.	Time and temperature control: quick chilling, reheating to 165°F (74°C).	Avoid unpasteurized milk and untreated water. Cook foods thoroughly. Wash hands thoroughly after handling raw poultry and meats.	Avoid cross-contamination. Cook ground beef to 155°F (68°C). Good personal hygiene.

Appendix H-2
Meat- and Egg-Cooking Regulations

FDA Model Food Code

Poultry	165°F (74°C)	Pork	150°F (66°C)
Ground beef	155°F (68°C)	Rare roast beef	130°F (54°C)
Egg	See recommendation	Reheating (except rare roast beef 130°F [54°C])	165°F (74°C)

Note: Refer to current websites for updated data.

American Egg Board—Egg Doneness Guidelines

Scrambled eggs, omelets, and frittatas	Cook until the eggs are thickened and no visible liquid egg remains.
Fried eggs	Cook both sides and increase the temperature the eggs reach, cook slowly and either baste the eggs, cover the pan with a lid, or turn the eggs. Cook until the whites are completely set and the yolks begin to thicken but are not hard.
Soft-cooked eggs	Bring eggs and water to a full, rolling boil. Turn off the heat, cover the pan, and let the eggs sit in the hot water about 4 to 5 minutes.
Poached eggs	Cook in gently simmering water until the whites are completely set and the yolks begin to thicken but are not hard, about 3 to 5 minutes. Avoid precooking and reheating poached eggs.
Baked goods, hard-cooked eggs	These will easily reach internal temperatures of more than 160°F when they are done. Note, however, that while *Salmonella* are destroyed when hard-cooked eggs are properly prepared, hard-cooked eggs can spoil more quickly than raw eggs. After cooking, cool hard-cooked eggs quickly under running cold water or in ice water. Avoid allowing eggs to stand in stagnant water. Refrigerate hard-cooked eggs in their shells promptly after cooling and use them within 1 week.
French toast, Monte Cristo sandwiches, crab or other fish cakes, quiches, stratas, baked custards, most casseroles	Cook or bake until a thermometer inserted at the center shows 160°F or a knife inserted near the center comes out clean. You may find it difficult to tell if a knife shows uncooked egg or melted cheese in some casseroles and other combination dishes that are thick or heavy and contain cheese—lasagna, for example. To be sure these dishes are done, check to see that a thermometer at the center of the dish shows 160°F. Also use a thermometer to help guard against uneven cooking due to hot spots and inadequate cooking due to varying oven temperatures.
Soft (stirred) custards, including cream pie, eggnog, and ice cream bases	Cook until thick enough to coat a metal spoon with a thin film and a thermometer shows 160°F or higher. After cooking, cool quickly by setting the pan in ice or cold water and stirring for a few minutes. Cover and refrigerate to chill thoroughly, at least 1 hour.
Soft (pie) meringue	Bake a 3-egg-white meringue spread on a hot, fully cooked pie filling in a preheated 350°F oven until the meringue reaches 160°F, about 15 minutes. For meringues using more whites, bake at 325°F (or a lower temperature) until a thermometer registers 160°F, about 25 to 30 minutes (or more). The more egg whites, the lower the temperature and the longer the time you need to cook the meringue through without excessive browning. Refrigerate meringue-topped pies until serving. Return leftovers to the refrigerator.

Courtesy: American Egg Board.

Appendix I
Heat Transfer

- **Radiation.** Energy waves travel through space and heat the surface of food (broiling, toasting).
- **Conduction.** Heat is transferred from molecule to molecule (pan or burner).
- **Convection.** Warmed air or water rises, creating currents that heat surface of food (air in oven, liquid in pan).
- **Microwave.** Electromagnetic waves penetrate food and attract and repel molecules.

Most foods are heated by a combination of heat transfer methods. The photographs below show how heat is transferred in a potato. The lightest area indicates the hottest part of the potato.

HEATING FOODS BY MICROWAVE

Microwaves are high-frequency electromagnetic waves and, like radio broadcast waves, do not break chemical bonds (unlike ultraviolet light, x-rays, and gamma rays). When produced by magnetron in a microwave oven, they penetrate the food ¾ to 1 inch (1.9 to 2.54 cm). The microwaves oscillate or alternate millions of times each second, and in doing so, attract and repel the polarized molecules in the food. The molecules in the food vibrate and create ***friction,*** which produces the ***heat energy*** that cooks the food.

A given amount of microwave energy is emitted by the magnetron, and this is divided among the foods placed in the oven. Doubling the amount of food placed in the oven ***nearly*** doubles the heating time. Areas of food not reached by the microwaves, as well as the containers, eventually are heated by ***conduction*** from the food heated by microwaves.

CAUTION! DO NOT OPERATE OVEN WHEN EMPTY!! DO NOT OPERATE OVEN IF DOOR IS DAMAGED!!

A. Factors affecting cooking times (Olson and Olson 1979):
- Temperature of food—frozen foods should be defrosted on low settings, prior to cooking; refrigerated food requires more time than the same room-temperature food.

- Density—denser foods require longer cooking
- Moisture—more moisture requires longer cooking (more heat)
  - 75%–90% (most heat): vegetable soups, casserole
  - 50%–60% (less heat): meat, poultry, fish
  - 20%–35% (least heat): breads, cakes
- Sugar and fat—more requires less cooking time
- Shape—thin slices cook faster than thick, chunky foods; round shapes cook more evenly than square or rectangular shapes.

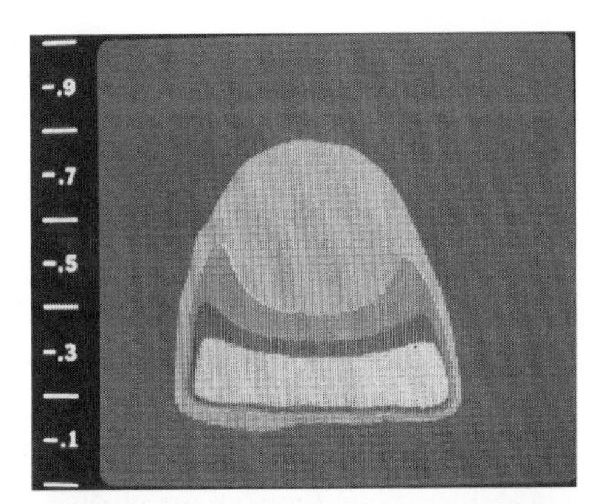

Range Top. After 8 Minutes, Heat has been Conducted from Bottom, but the Large Top Area of Potato is Uncooked.

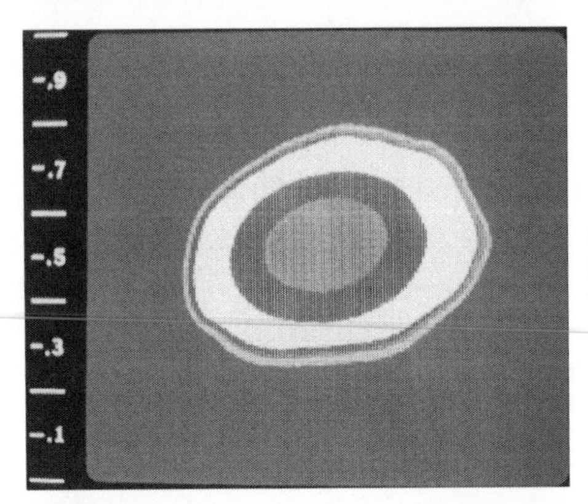

Oven. After 15 Minutes, the Heat from Surface is being Conducted to Interior; the Center is Uncooked.

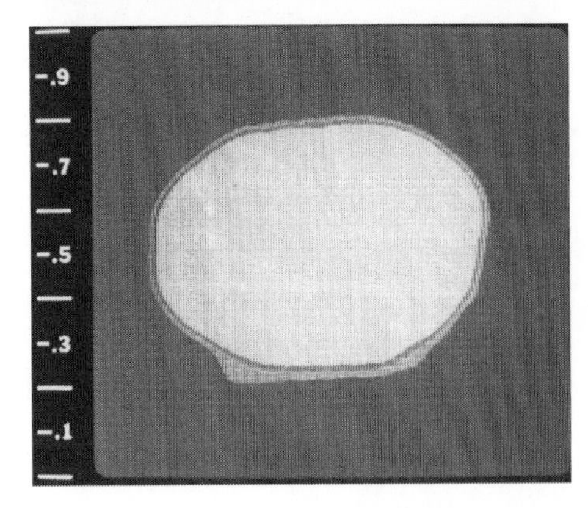

Microwave. After 4 Minutes, the Potato is Heated Throughout by Microwave Radiation and Conduction.

Courtesy: General Electric Co.

B. Utensils used in microwave ovens

- **May use**: Paper towels (caution with food contact by secondhand, recycled paper), plastic wrap (although no criteria for "microwave safe" are established), wax paper, glass and glass–ceramic, pottery, or china with no metallic contents, trim, or glaze.
- To test *if uncertain:* Place 1 cup (240 mL) water in glass and put it on or in a dish to be tested. Microwave 1 minute on HIGH. If water becomes hot, dish is safe (not absorbing microwave energy), but if *dish* is hot, do not use.
- **Avoid**: Metal pans, thermometers, skewers, foil trays, Corning Centura, Melamine dishes. Plastics vary in their ability to withstand microwave energy.

C. Browning

- Microwaving is moist heat cooking; therefore, browning is difficult to achieve, unless a browning utensil, special browning unit, or broiler is used in conjunction with microwaves.
- Many microwave recipes add special toppings to improve surface appearance:
  - *Quick breads, yeast breads*—toasted seeds, nuts or coconut, cinnamon sugar, herb seasonings
  - *Meats*—soup mixes, sauces such as soy or barbeque, browning and seasoning; crushed chips, or seasoned crumbs, paprika; microwave preparations to shake on
  - *Casseroles*—toasted breadcrumbs, cheese, sauces, fried dry onion rings, etc.

For consumer information on microwave oven radiation, consult Consumer Service Department of specific oven manufacturers or write: Microwave Ovens, HFX-28, Bureau of Radiological Health, Food and Drug Administration, Rockville, Maryland 20857; your state health department; or your local FDA office.

Reference

Olson, W. and R. Olson. 1979. *Heating Prepared Foods in Microwave Ovens.* North Central Regional Extension Publ. No. 72. Agricultural Extension Service, University of Minnesota.

Appendix J
Symbols for Measurements and Weights

A. Abbreviations

t or tsp = teaspoon	pk. = peck	oz. = ounce	g = gram
T or tbsp = tablespoon	pt. = pint	lb. = pound	kg = kilogram
c = cup	qt. = quart	fl. = fluid	mL = milliliter
bu. = bushel	gal. = gallon	fd = few drops	L = liter

B. Measurement Equivalents

(for laboratory use)

1 tbsp = 100 drops = 15 mL = 3 tsp	1 cup = 16 tbsp = 8 fl. oz. = 237 mL (240 mL) = ½ pt.	1 qt. = 4 cups = 32 fl. oz. = 2 pt. = 946.2 mL
1 gal. = 4 qt. = 3.8 L	1 kilo = 1000 g = 2.2 lb.	1 lb. = 16 oz. = 453.6 g (454 g) = 0.45 kg
1 g = 0.035 oz. = 1000 mg	1 oz. = 28.35 g (28 g) 3½ oz. = 100 g	

C. Temperature Conversions

$$°F = (°C + 32) \times 9/5$$
$$°C = (°F - 32) \times 5/9$$

Example:

$$144°F \text{ to } ?\ °C = (144°F - 32) \times 5/9$$
$$= 112°F \times 5/9$$
$$= 62°C$$

Appendix K
Notes on Test for Presence of Ascorbic Acid

Most measurements of ascorbic acid are based on its oxidation–reduction properties. When a substance *loses* hydrogen atoms or electrons, it is *oxidized*. The substance *gaining* the electrons is reduced. Carbon atoms 2 and 3 of ascorbic acid easily lose their hydrogen atoms to appropriate substances, forming dehydroascorbic acid.

C = O | C = O
C − OH | C = O
C − OH O | C = O O
H − C | H − C
HO − C − H | HO − C − H
CH_2OH | CH_2OH

$$\xrightarrow{-2H} \quad \xleftarrow[+2H]{}$$

Ascorbic acid (reduced form) | Dehydroascorbic acid (oxidized form)

For the test, a specific dye, 2,6-dichlorophenolindo-phenol, is used. It is purplish-blue in oxidized form, changing to light pink or becoming colorless when it is reduced. When solutions of ascorbic acid and the dye are reacted, the ascorbic acid gives up its hydrogen atoms to the dye. Ascorbic acid is oxidized and the dye is reduced. The reaction is indicated by change in color of the dye as shown below:

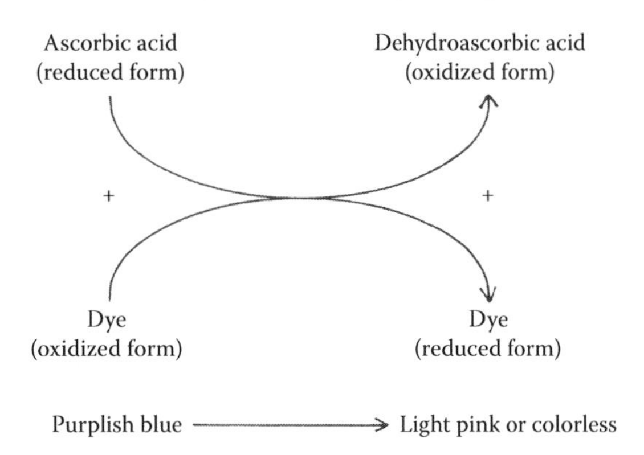

Other substances such as some sugars can also react with the dye. This test used with the foods suggested is a crude indicator of ascorbic acid concentration and the changes it undergoes during processing treatments.

Appendix L-1
Cooking Terms[1]

Bake: To cook in an oven or oven-type appliance. Covered or uncovered containers may be used.

Barbecue: To roast slowly on a spit or rack over coals or under a gas broiler flame or electric broiler unit, usually basting with a highly seasoned sauce. The term is commonly applied to foods cooked in or served with barbecue sauce.

Baste: To moisten food while cooking by pouring over it melted fat, drippings, or other liquid.

Blanch: To heat for a short period of time in boiling water or steam (precook).

Boil: To cook in water, or liquid sauce, at boiling temperature (212°F at sea level; 100°C). Bubbles rise continually and break on the surface.

Braise: To cook slowly in a moist atmosphere. The cooking is done in a tightly covered pot or pan with little or no added liquid. Meat may be browned in a small amount of fat before braising.

Broil: To cook uncovered by direct heat on a rack placed under the source of heat or over an open fire.

Pan broil: To cook in lightly greased or ungreased heavy pan on top of range. Fat is poured off as it accumulates, food does not fry.

Caramelize: To heat sugar or food containing sugar until a brown color and characteristic flavor develop.

Cream: To work a food or a combination of foods until soft and creamy, using a spoon, paddle, or other implement. Most often applied to fat or a mixture containing fat, for example, shortening and sugar.

Cut in: To distribute solid fat into dry ingredients using two knives or a pastry blender.

Fold: To combine two mixtures, or two ingredients such as beaten egg white and sugar, by cutting down gently through one side of the mixture with a spatula or other implement, bringing the spatula along the bottom of the mixture, and then folding over. This motion is repeated until the mixture is well blended.

Fricassee: To braise individual pieces of meat, poultry, or game in a little liquid—water, broth, or sauce.

Fry: To cook in fat without water or cover.

Pan-fry or sauté: To cook in a small amount of fat (a few tablespoons [or 45 mL] or more, up to ½ inch [1.25 cm]) in a fry pan.

Deep-fry or French-fry: To cook in a deep kettle, in enough fat to cover or float food.

Grill: To cook uncovered over an open fire or burner, griddle, or barbeque.

Knead: To press, stretch, and fold dough or similar mixture to make it smooth. During kneading, bread dough becomes elastic, fondant becomes smooth and satiny.

---

[1] Adapted by permission from *Family Fare,* Home and Garden Bulletin No. 1, USDA, 1973.

Marinate: To let foods stand in a liquid (usually mixture of oil with vinegar or lemon juice) to add flavor or make more tender.
Pare: To remove skins or peel from fruit or vegetable; peel.
Parboil: To boil until partly cooked.
Poach: To cook gently in liquid at simmering temperature so that the food retains its shape.
Pot-roast: To cook large pieces of meat by braising.
Pressure cook: To cook food in water and or steam in a pressure saucepan or canner at temperatures above 212°F (100°C).
Reconstitute: To restore concentrated foods to their original state; for example, to restore frozen concentrated orange juice to liquid form by adding water.
Rehydrate: To soak or cook to make dehydrated foods take up the water they lost during drying.
Roast: To bake in hot air (usually oven) without water to cover.
Sauté: To brown lightly in fat.
Scald: To heat liquid to about 149°F (65°C).
Simmer: To cook in liquid just below the boiling point, at a temperature of 185–210°F (85–98°C). Bubbles form slowly and break below the surface.
Steam: To cook food in steam, without pressure. Food is placed on a rack or a perforated pan over boiling water in a covered container.
Stew: To cook, covered, at simmering temperature, in a small amount of liquid.
Stir, blend, mix: To combine several ingredients to effect an even distribution throughout.
Whip: To beat rapidly to incorporate air.

Appendix L-2
Cuisine Terminology[2]

A

Adobo sauce: A thick, dark-red sauce native to Mexico, made from ground chiles mixed with spices and vinegar. Canned chipotles (smoked-dried jalapenos) are usually packed in adobo sauce.

Agneau: Lamb.

Al dente: Italian for "to the tooth," ***al dente*** describes pasta and other foods that are cooked just until they resist slightly when chewed—not undercooked or overdone.

Albumin: A water-soluble protein found in vegetables, bones, meat, and egg whites. Albumin coagulates as it is heated, collecting impurities as it moves—this is the scum on a stock. Rapid boiling destroys its ability to collect impurities, resulting in a cloudy stock.

À la carte: Individual items ordered from a menu.

À la mode: Dish topped with ice cream.

Amandine: With almonds.

Aromatics: Various spices, plant ingredients, or herbs (parsley, bay leaf, ginger, garlic, onion) that enhance and impart flavor to food.

Aubergine: Eggplant.

Au gratin: With cheese. Creamed with eggs, milk, or stock, covered with bread crumbs and cheese, then browned.

B

Baked Alaska: A cake or ice cream, covered with meringue, then browned.

Baste or mop: To moisten food while cooking with a liquid (melted fat, pan dripping, sauce, or other liquid). This keeps the meat, and other foods, from drying out and encourages color and flavor. A spoon, brush, bulb baster, or miniature mop can be used.

Bloom: Pale gray film, streaks, or blotches that appear on the surface of chocolate when the cocoa butter separates and forms crystals (usually as a result of storing in too warm a place). Blooming does not affect flavor or cooking properties.

Boeuf: Beef.

Bouquet garni: A bunch of herbs ties together or placed in a cheesecloth bundle. This allows the herbs to be easily removed from food before it is served. The classic herbs used in a bouquet garni are thyme, parsley, and bay leaf.

[2] Compiled from ***Cuisine At Home*** magazine and other references. Some of these definitions are protected by copyright owned by August Home Publishing Company and are used with specific permission of the publisher. They originally appeared in ***Cuisine At Home*** magazine. For more information about ***Cuisine At Home*** magazine, go to www.CuisineAtHome.com.

Break/separate: When two or more ingredients fail to hold together in one uniform state. Hollandaise, for example, can break or separate from a smooth sauce into one that is oily and curdled-looking.

Butterfly: To split food down the center, cutting almost through. The halves are fanned open and laid flat to cook. The fan resembles a butterfly.

C

Canapé: Open hors d'oeuvre—cracker, sandwich, or/spread on vegetable.

Canard: Duck.

Caramelization: All meat and vegetables contain some sugar (in the form of carbohydrates). Under intense dry heat, as in roasting or sautéing, these sugars break down. The result is the brown color and rich flavor called caramelization.

Champignon: Mushroom.

Chiffonade: French word meaning "made of rags." It refers to thin strips or shreds of vegetables and herbs. Several leaves are stacked on top of one another and rolled tightly like a cigar. Thin slices are made across the leaves while holding the roll tightly.

Chili vs. Chile: Chili refers to the dish. Chile is the Spanish spelling, used when referring to the fruit of the chile plant. An exception to this rule is chili pepper, which refers to the chile used to make chili.

Chitlins: Also called chitterlings, chitlins are the small intestines of freshly slaughtered hogs. They are simmered until tender, and may be used in soups, or battered and fried after boiling.

Chowder: A thick soup of clam, seafood, or vegetables.

Concassée: A term whose root word means to roughly chop or pound a food. Concassée is usually made from chopped tomatoes.

Crème fraîche: A tangy thickened cream, of French origin, similar in taste and texture to sour cream. In France, pasteurization is not required. Therefore, the cream contains bacteria that thicken it naturally. Unlike sour cream, crème fraîche is used in sauces and soups because it can be boiled without breaking.

Crepe: French pancake—typically filled with a sweetened ingredient or creamed main dish.

Cryovac: A registered trademark for a process in which meat is sealed in plastic, and all the air is removed by a vacuum pump.

D

Dash: Very small quantity; of a teaspoon quantity.

Deglaze: The process of removing browned bits of food from the bottom of the pan. It is done by heating a small amount of liquid in the pan (usually wine or stock), and stirring to loosen. This mixture is a great base for making a sauce.

De jour: Foods "of the day" offered by a restaurant.

Devein: To remove the dark brownish-black vein that runs down the back of a shrimp. The vein is really the intestinal tract of the shrimp. In smaller shrimp, the vein can be eaten, but in larger shrimp, the vein contains grit and should be removed.

Dock: To pierce pastry dough before baking to allow steam to escape and prevent blistering of the dough.

Dredge: To lightly coat food with dry ingredients like flour, cornmeal, or bread crumbs. A usual preparation for frying to help brown the food.

E

Egg wash: Egg yolk, white, or whole egg beaten with a small amount of water or milk. The mixture is then brushed over breads and pastries before baking to give them color and sheen.
Entrée: Main dish.

F

Farci: Stuffed.
Florentine: With spinach.

G

Glaze: 1. A 90% reduction of stock. 2. A thin glossy coating applied to foods. A reduction or aspic can cover savory foods. Anything from melted chocolate to thin icings can cover pastries and cakes. Verb: To apply a thin, shiny coating to food.
Grenouille: Frog.

H

Homard: Lobster.
Hors d'oeuvre: Appetizer—hot or cold, served after soup.
Hydroponic: A technique for growing vegetables in nutrient-enriched water instead of soil.

I

Infusion: The extraction of flavor from a food in a hot liquid (below the boiling point). Usually refers to teas and coffees, but can also apply to cooking (like the pistachio cream or olive oils that are infused with herbs).

J

Jambon: Ham.
Julienne: Foods that are cut into thin, match-stick strips.

K

Kalamata olive: Olive native to Greece, almond-shaped with a dark eggplant color and a pungent, fruity flavor. Kalamata olives are often split before being packing in oil or vinegar to allow the marinade to soak into the flesh.

L

Legume: Vegetable. A pod, such as that of a pea or bean that splits into two halves with seeds attached to the pod.

Lyonaise: With onions, highly seasoned.

M

Menu: A small detailed list. What is offered and served.

Mesclun: A French term meaning "mixed." It refers to a salad comprising small, delicate salad leaves and herbs.

Milling: The mechanical processing of grinding, cracking, and/or removing the hull, bran, or germ from whole grains.

Mirepoix: A mixture of diced carrots, onions, celery, and herbs sautéed in butter. Mirepoix is used to season sauces, soups, and stews. It is also used as a bed to braise meats and fish.

Mother sauces: A French concept that classifies all sauces into five foundation sauces called "mother" or "grand sauces." From these five sauces, all sauces can be made. They are: 1. demi-glace or brown; 2. velouté or blond; 3. béchamel or white; 4. hollandaise or butter; 5. tomato or red.

Mount: A technique where small pieces of cold, unsalted butter are whisked into a sauce just before serving. Mounting gives sauces texture and flavor as well as a glossy look.

MSG: Monosodium glutamate; looks like fine salt. It has no pronounced flavor of its own, but can intensify the flavor of savory foods, and is used as a flavor enhancer.

N

Nonreactive pan or bowl: Any nonporous material that does not impart a flavor or alter a color in food. This includes glass, stainless steel, glazed ceramic, or enamel.

O

O'Brien: With added pepper, onion, and pimento.

Oxidation: A chemical reaction that occurs when a substance is exposed to oxygen. The oxygen reacts with elements in the substance to change it. The color of food is often affected, as when cut apples turn brown.

P

Parboil: Partial cooking of a food in boiling or simmering liquid. Similar to blanching, but the cooking time is longer.

Pinch: 1/16 of a teaspoon quantity.

Pita: A Middle Eastern flat bread, also called pocket bread. The round loaves are easily split in half, which makes them perfect for stuffing with sandwich fillings. Pita are found frozen or fresh at most markets.

Pith: The soft, white membrane that lies between the peel and the pulp of a citrus fruit. It has a bitter flavor.

Polenta: An Italian cornmeal mush that is often cooled and then fried, grilled, broiled, or baked.

Proof: In short, swelling. Yeast proofs when it swells and becomes bubbly. A dough proofs when it swells and rises to twice its original size.

Prosciutto: This "ham" is Italy's gift to the food world. The cities of Parma and San Daniele (where it is mainly produced) argue over whose is better. Its production is a secret. It is first seasoned and salt-cured (but not smoked), then air-dried, pressed, and sold thinly sliced. The best hams are aged 18 to 24 months.

Pulse: The edible seeds of pod-bearing plants such as beans or peas.

Q

Quadrillage: From the French word ***quadrille***, meaning marked with squares or rectangles. In cooking, it refers to the square charred marks that are the result of a grill's hot grate "branding" the food.

Queso fresco: A white Mexican cheese, similar in flavor and texture to feta. It softens when heated, but does not melt. It is best crumbled on top of dishes like tamales and tacos.

R

Ramekin: A small ceramic or earthenware baking dish. The bottom should be rough (unglazed) to prevent suction from forming in water bath between ramekin and pan.

Reduce: Applied to cooking, this means to boil a liquid until its volume is reduced by evaporation. This thickens the liquid and intensifies the flavor.

Reduction: A process used to increase and intensify the flavor of a liquid. This is done by rapidly boiling a liquid to decrease its volume through evaporation. This concentrates the flavor, so season a reduction after it is made—not before.

Refresh/shock: To submerge a cooked food, usually a vegetable, in cold water to cool it quickly and stop further cooking.

Render: The melting of animal fat over low heat so it separates from any connective tissue. This tissue turns crisp and brown (known as crackling) and the clarified (clear) fat is further processed by straining. To cook fatty meats, such as bacon or spare ribs, until the fat melts.

Rennet: A coagulating enzyme usually from the stomach lining of young animals (some can come from plants) that aids in curdling milk or separating curds from whey.

Resting: Heat drives meat's juices from the surface when it cooks. Letting meat "rest" before slicing lets these juices seep back toward the surface (liquids always take the path of least resistance). The result is a more flavorful piece of meat.

Ribbon: When a sauce thickens enough that, when lifted, it falls in wide bands. Also, when sauce is thick enough that while stirred with a whisk, it leaves trails that expose the bottom of the pan or mixing bowl.

Ricer: A kitchen gadget that looks like a big garlic press. This device, also called a potato ricer, forces cooked foods like turnips and potatoes through tiny holes, so that they resemble rice.

S

Sashimi: Sliced raw fish that is usually served with daikon radish, pickled ginger, wasabi, and soy sauce. It is usually the first course in a Japanese meal. Because it is served raw, only the freshest and highest-quality fish should be used for sashimi.

Season: To coat a pan or other metal cooking surface (not nonstick) with oil and then heat it. This prevents sticking by sealing tiny pits in the metal. Soap and water can negate this effect.

Springform pan: A round pan with tall, straight sides that "unbuckle" from a removable bottom, most often used for tortes and cheesecakes. Allows a cake to be easily unmolded and still retain its shape.

Sushi: A Japanese specialty based on steamed rice flavored with sweetened rice vinegar. There is a wide variety of sushi, but most include slices of raw fish placed on top of this rice. Another type includes vegetables enclosed in a sushi rice, then rolled in seaweed sheets (nori) and sliced.

Sweat: When foods, usually vegetables, are cooked over low heat in a small amount of fat (usually butter), drawing out juices to remove rawness and develop flavor.

T

Table d'hôte: "Table of the host." All courses on the menu sold at one price as opposed to à la carte.

Tamarind: Fruit of a tall shade tree native to Asia and North Africa. The large brown pods contain small seeds and sweet-sour pulp. This pulp is a common flavoring in Indian and Middle Eastern cuisines; use like lemon juice.

Temper: To slowly add a hot liquid to eggs or other foods to gradually raise their temperature without making them curdle.

Tempura: Japanese batter-dipped, deep-fried fish or vegetables. Cold water in the batter allows food to steam within hot oil-sealed batter. Creates a puffy coating and makes food cook faster.

Timbale: A high-sided, drum-shaped mold that can taper toward the bottom. The food baked in the mold is usually a custard-based dish that is unmolded before serving.

Tripe: From the lining of beef cattle stomachs. Smooth or flat tripe is from the first stomach, and honeycomb and pocket tripe are from the second stomach. Tripe is tough, requiring long cooking in stews or casseroles.

Turmeric: The root of a tropical plant related to ginger with a bitter flavor and bright orange-yellow color. Turmeric adds flavor and color to many foods, including American-style yellow mustard.

Z

Zest: The zest is the colored portion of the skin (not the white pith) of citrus fruits. The aromatic oils in the citrus zest are what adds so much flavor to food. Use in cooked and raw foods.

Appendix M
Buying Guide[1]

VEGETABLES AND FRUITS

Note: A serving of a vegetable is ½ cup (120 mL) cooked vegetable unless otherwise noted. A serving of fruit is ½ cup (120 mL) fruit; 1 medium apple, banana, peach, or pear; or 2 apricots or plums. A serving of cooked fresh or dried fruit is ½ cup (120 mL) fruit and liquid.

Fresh Vegetables	Servings per lb. (454 g) as Purchased
Asparagus	3 or 4
Beans, lima[a]	2
Beans, snap	5 or 6
Beets, diced[b]	3 or 4
Broccoli	3 or 4
Brussels sprouts	4 or 5
Cabbage	
Raw, shredded	9 or 10
Cooked	4 or 5
Carrots	
Raw, diced, or shredded[b]	5 or 6
Cooked[b]	4
Cauliflower	3
Celery	
Raw, chopped, or diced	5 or 6
Cooked	4
Kale[c]	5 or 6
Okra	4 or 5
Onions, cooked	3 or 4
Parsnips[b]	4
Peas[a]	2
Potatoes	4
Spinach[d]	4
Squash, summer	3 or 4
Squash, winter	2 or 3
Sweet potatoes	3 or 4
Tomatoes, raw, diced, or sliced	4

[a] Bought in pod. [b] Bought without tops. [c] Bought untrimmed. [d] Bought prepackaged.

[1] Adapted from *Buying Food,* Home Economics Research Report No. 42 USDA, 1978.

Canned Vegetables	Servings per Can, 1 lb. (454 g)
Most vegetables	3 or 4
Greens, such as kale or spinach	2 or 3
Frozen Vegetables	**Servings per Package, 9 or 10 oz. (252–280 g)**
Asparagus	2 or 3
Beans, lima	3 or 4
Beans, snap	3 or 4
Broccoli	3
Brussels sprouts	3
Cauliflower	3
Corn, whole kernel	3
Kale	2 or 3
Peas	3
Spinach	2 or 3
Dry Vegetables	**Servings per lb. (454 g)**
Dry beans	11
Dry peas, lentils	10 or 11
Fresh Fruits	**Servings per Market Unit, A.P.**
Apples, bananas, peaches, pears, and plums	3 or 4/lb. (454 g)
Apricots; cherries, sweet; grapes, seedless	5 or 6/lb. (454 g)
Blueberries	4 or 5/pt. (480 mL)
Raspberries, strawberries	8 or 9/qt. (950 mL)
Frozen Fruit	**Servings per Package, 10–12 oz. (300–360 mL)**
Blueberries	3 or 4
Peaches	2 or 3
Raspberries	2 or 3
Strawberries	2 or 3
Canned Fruit	**Servings per Can, 1 lb. (454 g)**
Served with liquid	4
Drained	2 or 3
Dried Fruit	**Servings per Package, 8 oz. (224 g)**
Apples	8
Apricots	6
Mixed fruits	6
Peaches	7
Pears	4
Prunes	4 or 5

Meat Products

Meat Products	Size of Serving
Beef, ground	4 servings/lb (454 g)
Chicken breast halves	2.75 halves/lb. (454 g)
	1 half = 3 oz. (85 g)
Chicken thighs	4.5 thighs/lb. (454 g)
(cooked meat)	2 thighs = 3 oz. (85 g)

Cereals and Cereal Products

Cereals and Cereal Products	Size of Serving		Servings per lb. (454 g)
Flaked corn cereals	1 cup	240 mL	16
Other flaked cereals	¾ cup	180 mL	21
Puffed cereals	1 cup	240 mL	32–38
Cornmeal	½ cup	120 mL	22
Wheat cereals			
Coarse	½ cup	120 mL	16
Fine	½ cup	120 mL	20–27
Oatmeal	½ cup	120 mL	16
Hominy grits	½ cup	120 mL	20
Macaroni and noodles	½ cup	120 mL	17
Rice	½ cup	120 mL	16
Spaghetti	½ cup	120 mL	18
Flour (all purpose)	1 cup	240 mL	4
Cornmeal, dry	1 cup	240 mL	3

Miscellaneous

Miscellaneous	Cups per lb. (240 mL/454 g)
Hydrogenated fats	2½
Butter, margarine, lard	2
Oil	2
Cottage cheese	2
Granulated sugar	2
Brown sugar, packed	2
Confectioner's sugar	3½

Appendix N
Spice and Herb Chart

Herbs/Spices	Main Dish	Salads	Sauces	Vegetables
Spices				
Allspice	Beef pot roast, duck, turkey or chicken, fish	Fruit salad	Tomato	Beets
Cayenne	Beef, stews, chicken, seafood	All varieties except fruit	Meat, vegetable	All vegetables
Chili powder	Beef, hamburgers, meatloaf, chili con carne	Bean salad	Mexican type	Corn
Cloves	Pork, ham, boiled beef, pot roast		Tomato, sweet/sour	
Curry	Meat, fish, poultry, lamb, veal, fish or shrimp chowders	Chicken salad	Vegetable	Rice, creamed onions
Ginger	Pork, chicken	Fruit salad	Dessert	Squash
Mace	Poultry stuffing, veal	Fruit salad	Fish, poultry, veal	Potatoes
Dry mustard	Beef, hamburgers, chicken, tuna, egg	Chicken, egg, tuna, macaroni, potato	Fish, vegetable	Cabbage
Nutmeg	Chicken stew, beef stew, creamed dishes	Fruit salad	Dessert, fruit sauces; pudding	All vegetables except cabbage family
Paprika	Meat, fish, poultry, veal, creamed dishes	All except fruit salad	All gravies and sauces	All vegetables
Pepper	Meat, fish, poultry, veal	All except fruit salad	All gravies and sauces	All vegetables

(Continued)

Appendix N (cont'd)
Spice and Herb Chart

Herbs/Spices	Main Dish	Salads	Sauces	Vegetables
Herbs				
Basil	Tomato, egg, fish, chicken cacciatore, beef stew	Vegetable salads with marinades	Tomato	Cucumbers, green beans, zucchini
Chives	Creamed dishes, fish, eggs	Potato salad, green salad	Creamed type	Potatoes
Dill	Fish	Potato, vegetable	Creamed type	Green beans, cucumbers, cabbage, carrots
Marjoram	Italian type, tomato, beef, lamb, fish	Salad dressings	Tomato, brown	Broccoli, green beans, peas, eggplant
Oregano	Italian type, tomato, meatloaf, pork, veal, pot roast	Vegetable salads, marinades, bean salad, salad	Tomato, fish	Tomato, broccoli, zucchini, eggplant
Parsley	All	All except fruit salad	All except fruit	All
Rosemary	Beef, pork, fish, lamb		Vegetable, meat and fish gravies	Cauliflower, potatoes, turnips
Sage	Pork, poultry, goulash beef stew	Vegetable salads with marinades	Meat, chicken, pork gravies	Mushroom, broccoli, cabbage, onions, cauliflower
Thyme	Beef, pork, chicken, fish, beef stews, fish chowders, fish soups	Vegetable salads with marinades, salad dressings	Brown	Creamed onions
Tarragon	Eggs, poultry, fish	Salad dressings	Creamed type	Potatoes

Courtesy: Campbell Soup Company.

Appendix O
Plant Proteins

Meat, fish, eggs, and milk occupy a prominent place in the American diet. Although these foods are excellent sources of protein and several other nutrients, ***moderation*** of their consumption is advocated for several reasons. The recent U.S. *Dietary Guidelines* suggest moderation of intakes of total fat, saturated fat, and cholesterol. These animal protein sources contribute a significant portion of these substances to our diets. Further, production of animal protein is expensive. About 10 pounds of grain are required to produce 1 pound of meat. Accordingly, for the consumer, the price of animal foods is high. Shrinking food resources and rising food prices oblige us to question extensive use of animal foods to meet protein needs. Less expensive plant proteins can adequately meet protein needs if nutritional principles are clearly understood.

Recall that protein *per se* is not an essential nutrient. Rather, dietary protein provides amino acids and nitrogen. Thus, the protein value of a specific food depends on the total quantity of protein present and the quality of the amino acid pattern. At least 22 different amino acids are used in body processes. Some of these amino acids are synthesized by body cells from commonly available materials. Nine are called essential amino acids because the body cannot synthesize them from any materials. The nine essential amino acids are valine, lysine, threonine, leucine, isoleucine, tryptophan, phenylalanine, histidine, and the sulfur-containing amino acid, methionine. These nine must be obtained from food ***preformed, ready to use,*** and ***in appropriate amounts.*** Further, for efficient utilization, the body requires all nine essential amino acids to be ingested at about the same time. ***Protein quality*** of a single food is judged by its capacity to provide the essential amino acids in appropriate amounts.

Single foods differ in protein quality. The nutritive excellence of such foods as meat and milk is due to their complete amino acid pattern. For this reason, animal foods are said to have ***complete proteins.*** Gelatin is an exception to the usual high quality of animal foods; it is an ***incomplete protein*** because one essential amino acid is missing.

Many plant foods have substantial amounts of protein. Although the nine essential amino acids are present, some are not present in sufficient amounts. Thus, plant proteins are classed as ***partially complete.*** The most frequently limiting amino acids are lysine, threonine, tryptophan, and sulfur-containing amino acids. Individual foods differ as to their essential amino acid composition. These differences are summarized in Table O.1. Because threonine is generally adequate if needs for the other three are met, it is not included in the summary.

To meet body needs, it does not matter whether the essential amino acids come from a single food or from a combination of foods. The key to using plant proteins to meet protein needs is understanding

TABLE O.1

	Amino Acids	
Food Groups	Good Source of:	Poor Source of:
Legumes	Lysine	Tryptophan S-C[a]
Soybeans	Lysine[b]	S-C
Dry beans	Tryptophan[b] Lysine[b]	Tryptophan S-C
Nuts–Seeds	Tryptophan S-C	Lysine
Peanuts	Tryptophan	Lysine S-C
Sesame seed	Tryptophan S-C[b]	Lysine
Cereals–Grains	Tryptophan S-C	Lysine
Cornmeal	S-C	Lysine Tryptophan
Whole wheat flour	Tryptophan S-C	Lysine
Wheat germ	Lysine[b]	Tryptophan S-C
Rice	Tryptophan S-C	Lysine
Eggs	Lysine[b] Tryptophan[b] S-C[b]	
Meat, Fish, Poultry	Lysine[b] Tryptophan S-C	
Dairy	Lysine[b] Tryptophan[b] S-C[b]	

[a] S-C: sulfur-containing amino acids.

[b] Superior.

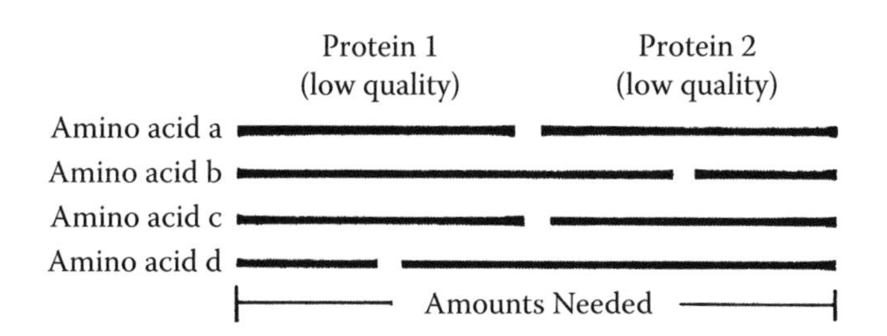

FIGURE O.1 Combining protein 1 and 2 provides good-quality protein.

their amino acid composition (see Table O.1). A few plant proteins, such as soy, have good amounts of the essential amino acids. Thus, by increasing the quantity of plant proteins like soy eaten at one time, essential amino acid needs can be met. Plant proteins can be combined with a small amount of animal protein or two or more plant proteins can be combined so there is mutual supplementation of the amino acids of the different foods. When two foods supplement each other in amino acid patterns, the combination gives greater protein quality than either could provide if eaten alone. This concept is illustrated in Figure O.1.

Because animal foods generally have a complete amino acid pattern, they complement most plant foods. Dairy foods are particularly effective complements of plant protein because they are good sources of lysine. A small amount of meat improves the protein quality of grains and legumes. Cereal and milk, macaroni and cheese, spaghetti and meatballs, peanut butter, and milk are examples of complementing plant foods with a small amount of animal food.

Combining two or more plant proteins to obtain high-quality protein depends on matching the amino acid strengths and weakness of individual foods. Nuts, seeds, and grains are generally low in lysine and relatively good in tryptophan and sulfur-containing amino acids. In general, legumes are good sources of lysine and poor sources of tryptophan and sulfur-containing amino acids. Exceptions to those generalizations are noted in Table O.1. With complementary combinations of plant foods, like rice and beans, the resulting amino acid pattern can be equal to animal foods. However, evaluation of total nutrient intake is important when plant foods are extensively substituted for animal foods. Particular attention should be given to amounts of vitamin D, B_{12}, riboflavin, and minerals provided in an all-vegetarian diet. Table O.1 provides a starting point for investigating various protein food combinations. More detailed information is given in the references cited below.

Use of plant foods as major protein sources is not a new concept. The traditional dishes of many cultures illustrate the concept's extensive application over the years. Currently, the ***Dietary Guidelines***, the world food shortages, and high food prices re-emphasize the value of plant proteins. Creative use of the principles of mutual supplementation not only spares animal foods and stretches the food dollar without sacrificing of protein quality but also opens up a range of new eating experiences.

References

Guthrie, H.A. 1989. *Introductory Nutrition,* 7th edition. St. Louis, MO: Times Mirror/Mosby College Publishing.
Lappé, F.M. 1991. *Diet for a Small Planet,* 20th edition. New York: Ballantine Books.
Robertson, L., C. Flinders, and B. Ruppenthal. 1986. *The New Laurel's Kitchen.* Berkeley, CA: Ten Speed Press.
Whitney, E.N. and S.R. Rolfes. 2008. *Understanding Nutrition*, 11th edition. Belmont, CA: Wadsworth.

Appendix P
Websites—Frozen Desserts[1]

A popular food product consumed year-round is frozen desserts. Frozen desserts include nondairy, lactose-free, soy, low-sugar, gluten-free, vegan, kosher, brand-name recipes, restaurant recipes, and so forth. Several websites are listed below.

www.baking911.com/frozen/
—Ice cream; freezies/smoothies/whips; frozen custard or French ice cream; frozen soufflé; frozen yogurt; fruit ice; gelato/gelati: granita (also granité) or ice; ice cream roulade (rolls); ice milk; Italian ice; mousse; novelties; parfait; popsickle; sherbet; sorbet; tofulati; tofuti; tofutti; quiescently frozen confection.

www.bhg.com—Better Homes and Gardens. Search Frozen Desserts.
www.cspinet.org/nah/6_98des.htm Center for Science in the Public Interest comparisons

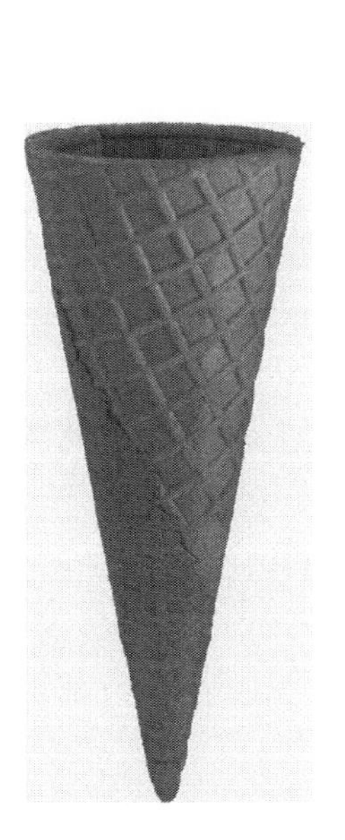

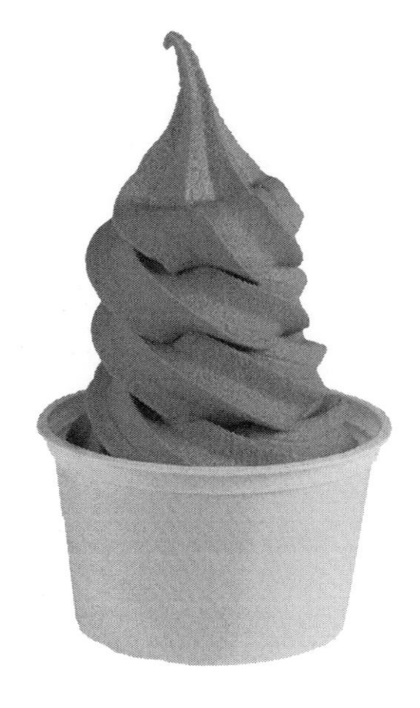

Courtesy: SYSCO® Incorporated.

[1] Other commercial and noncommercial websites may be utilized.

An environmentally friendly book printed and bound in England by www.printondemand-worldwide.com

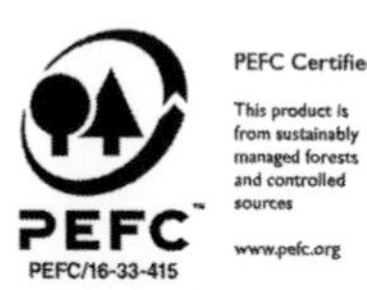

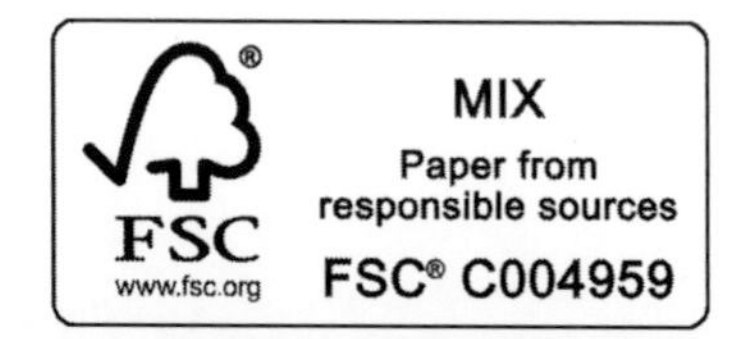